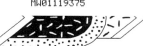

MW01119375

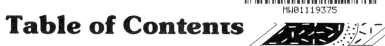

Table of Contents

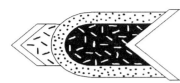 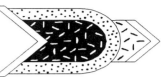

Preface

Leisure is the Art of Life. If what you do is drawn by your own hand and crafted with love, a stick figure or a lump of clay will meet your needs better than stealing a Picasso.

I get excited each time one of my children bounces a basketball, swings on the swing, does a cartwheel, draws a picture, plays catch, rolls a ball, works on a craft project, reads a story, writes a poem and on and on. I get excited because I know they are functioning on a high leisure level and that this participation is in a healthy direction.

When a person who is unhealthy participates in similar activities, I get excited, too, because I know that the person is also making steps to improve his/her life by participating on a high leisure level. Recreational therapy is a primary therapy in the mental health field and can be one of the most important psychiatric interventions in helping those with mental illness.

For those of you who work in Rehab or Long Term Care, I hope you experience the same excitement in seeing your patients or residents recover the ability to participate in recreation activities again after illness or injury. In MR/DD you can see your clients learn healthy recreation skills, perhaps for the first time.

The **Leisure Step Up Workbook** is a comprehensive guide, taking the participant on an eleven step journey to a healthy leisure lifestyle. It contains an assessment, a leisure plan, leisure education, self awareness, leisure planning and leisure participation. Completion of the workbook will help to bring about a desired change in the participant's leisure lifestyle and in the individual.

Our leisure time is of the utmost importance since it represents a freedom of choice that is different from our choices in other facets of life. That is what makes our free time so important. We make our choices and then we receive our consequences accordingly. It is important to choose wisely!

Note on terminology:

The **Leisure Step Up** can be used with a wide variety of populations and in a wide variety of settings. While it is most appropriate for people with psychological problems, it can also be used with people with physical or developmental disabilities or with people in nursing homes. Because the people being served may be called patients, clients or residents depending on the setting, this book will use the term **participant** to refer to people who are working on the **Leisure Step Up** program. Regardless of what other things are happening in their lives, when it comes to leisure, everything depends on participation.

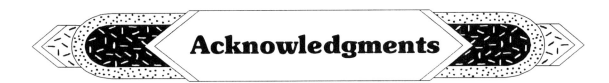

Acknowledgments

A note of thanks to my wife Cathy and my three children, Jonathan (Jono), Laney (Na Na) and Caitlyn (K-K) for our wonderful shared leisure time together. Also for the leisure time given to me to write and share this material with you.

To those in the Mental Health field who have shared and been my friend for both personal and professional growth, I give thanks.

A special thanks to Katherine Gomez who was greatly supportive in giving of herself in typing the original manuscript and for an unrelenting positive attitude.

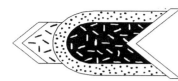 **Introduction**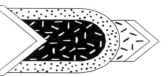

Leisure is more than just what we do in our "free time". It is through leisure that we are able to provide ourselves with the physical exercise we need, to develop and practice the skills required for interacting with others, to assimilate new ideas or to figure out where the ideas that we already have actually fit into our lives. Even more, leisure provides for us a quality of life which can move us to greater and greater levels of health and happiness. It can help bring contentment and peace to our lives. When we do not have these basic skills and experiences either through lack of knowing we need to or through other barriers, we risk developing or complicating illnesses or disabilities. Like the need for balanced nutrition, we need a balanced leisure lifestyle to promote and maintain our basic health.

As therapists, many of the people that we work with have unbalanced leisure lifestyles. This unbalance may be one of the reasons the person needs medical or psychiatric treatment or it may be secondary to the person's medical diagnosis. In either case, the people we work with are not likely to have the ability to correct the imbalance in their leisure lifestyle without some assistance, either in the form of guidance and intervention from a therapist or maybe with just a little help from a "map" or a "how to" book.

To be able to learn a complex skill, all of us need to learn the different components of that skill, mastering each, to some degree, along the way. For without the acquisition of skills related to each of the components of a complex skill, we may never be able to be truly independent in the skill itself. Acquiring and maintaining a healthy leisure lifestyle is a very complex skill — one that we must constantly work on if we want to maintain a balance.

Why will it be a constant struggle to maintain the balance, even after we have mastered a healthy balanced leisure lifestyle? Because our world changes. Our body grows older, our personal needs change. We may have a change in geographic location which requires us to develop a whole new support system and leisure network. Or we may lose our closest friend or lover. Each change in our lives requires us to adjust our leisure lifestyle to help maintain health. The Greeks have an appropriate saying, "The same person never steps in the same river twice."

We can only make the adjustments we need to make if we have the skills and knowledge to be self-directed in our leisure lifestyle. The recreational therapist cannot always, nor should s/he always, be there to help us adjust.

The lack of a healthy leisure lifestyle is evident enough, whether the lifestyle is the primary cause of the disability or illness or whether it is as a result of the disability or illness. Individuals who rely on alcohol or drugs for leisure do not have a healthy leisure lifestyle. Individuals with a traumatic brain injury are at a significantly greater risk of acquiring a first time drug or alcohol dependency if they have not (re)developed a healthy leisure balance. The examples are numerous. And while the ability to develop the complex skills of finding and maintaining a healthy leisure lifestyle is a difficult task, the steps to do so are, luckily, pretty clear and straight forward.

This book helps the therapist teach the participant the complex skills for developing and maintaining a healthy leisure lifestyle. By taking the required steps of learning and presenting them to the participant in a developmental sequence, the participant will have a greater chance of having success. The **Leisure Step Up** has broken the steps down into a developmental sequence, with instructions for the therapist and worksheets for the participant. The participant will not always have the therapist with him/her. By working through the worksheets once with the assistance of a trained therapist and then having the worksheets to refer to after discharge, the participant has a tool to help him/her through the changes in his/her life.

The skill to take responsibility for his/her own healthy leisure lifestyle is also likely to have a positive effect on the participant's ability to take responsibility for his/her own healthy lifestyle in general. The skills to acquire and maintain a healthy leisure lifestyle are basically the same skills required to maintain a healthy lifestyle — with just a little transference.

The development of these skills is not a straight path from the "bottom" to the "top". It is more like a helix — a continually spiraling, always moving path. The participant identifies a need for change, goes through the steps to master the needed change, achieves the change to some degree and then starts all over again as s/he realizes that there is another need for change or modification to meet life's events. It is hoped that with each move the participant will be able to achieve a greater level of a healthy leisure lifestyle or at least acquire knowledge and skills which will help with the next quest.

What is this "healthy leisure lifestyle" that we all should be trying to attain? This book is based on the *Leisure Level Model* first conceptualized by Nash[1]. In all, there are nine levels in this model — at the bottom, three "negative" levels; in the middle, one neutral level; and at the top, five positive levels. People will tend to function in more than one level at any given time. The two important questions in this model are *Which leisure levels can the person achieve independently?* and *Does the person choose to function at levels which lead to a healthy and satisfying leisure lifestyle?*

As the participant spirals through the acquisition of a healthier leisure lifestyle, s/he will become aware of barriers to a healthy leisure lifestyle and will gain the knowledge and skills necessary to break through the barriers. S/he will learn how to participate at higher positive levels of leisure. Each time through the program, s/he can identify and get through more barriers and so be able to participate in more and more activities at a higher leisure level.

---

[1]Nash, J. B. 1953. **Philosophy of Recreation and Leisure**. Dubuque, Iowa: Wm. C. Brown Company.

What is the Leisure Step Up?

The **Leisure Step Up** is an eleven step process which helps the participant gain the skills and knowledge s/he needs to progress toward a healthy leisure lifestyle. It does this in a developmentally appropriate sequence, giving participants positive direction for solving problems, meeting basic needs and leading a healthy leisure lifestyle. Since learning about and experiencing the positive aspects of leisure is not just a cognitive exercise, this book uses both written work, instruction from the therapist and actual practice in the use of appropriate leisure skills. The program itself has both an instructor's manual and a workbook. The therapist will need to draw upon the opportunities and resources within the participant's community to help them further develop and practice leisure skills.

This book teaches the foundation of a healthy leisure lifestyle. It teaches the participant the importance of leisure, that it is his/her choice and responsibility for what s/he does during leisure time. The participant gains the ability to overcome barriers that have hampered his/her ability to choose a healthy leisure lifestyle in the past.

Background

The **Leisure Step Up** will assist the recreational therapist in the step by step process of assessment, problem identification, goal setting, educating and actual experience (participation) in leisure. The program also helps the participant experience problem solving in a supportive environment and in addressing health maintenance issues specific to their situation. Many recreational therapists find that they know what kind of information and skills their participants need but have no formal program to help their participants develop that information or skill base. This book is a formal program for participants which provides a progressive, systematic approach to the development of the basic knowledge and skills required to maintain a healthy leisure lifestyle.

The **Leisure Step Up** program has been used since 1991 with a variety of participant populations including:

- Adults admitted to Behavioral Medicine Programs
- Adolescents admitted to Behavioral Medicine Programs
- Adults admitted to Drug and Alcohol Treatment Programs
- Adolescents admitted to Drug and Alcohol Treatment Programs
- Adults in Leisure and Wellness Education
- Health Care staff (inservice and continuing education programs)

In hospitalization and patient care lengths of stays have decreased, programs are going to out patient and partial care and participant to staff ratios and paper work are increasing. The therapist does not have time to "hold the participant's hand" through the entire process of acquiring a knowledge base and during each leisure experience. Nor would "holding the participant's hand" necessarily be therapeutic — the participant needs to have the supportive experience of taking responsibility for his/her own healthy leisure development. By providing "homework" while the participant is in treatment, the therapist can monitor how well the participant does with limited supervision and support. This provides a clearer picture of how well the participant is likely to perform once s/he is discharged. The participant enjoys completing assignments on his/her own while the therapist remains instrumental in offering therapeutic intervention.

Finally, the general public is frequently lacking in the understanding of the benefits of healthy positive leisure participation and the consequences of unhealthy leisure participation. The **Leisure Step Up** can assist in the educational process of the community as a whole.

The Program

The program has three parts. The first part, consisting of three of the eleven steps, helps the participant establish the foundation for a healthy leisure lifestyle. It helps him/her realize that s/he has a need related to leisure and then teaches the initial steps to resolve the need.

Beginning with Step 1 the participant has an information handout and a quick recreational therapy assessment. This helps him/her realize that there may be a problem (or barrier) to a healthy, leisure lifestyle. The therapist can use the information from this step to help plan work in later steps.

Step 2 walks the participant through the process of identifying a problem then offers initial direction for solving the problem through healthy leisure participation. The problem does not have to be leisure-based, but the solution is. For example, the problem could be low self-esteem caused by domestic violence. The solution could be using leisure activities to increase self-esteem.

Step 3 helps provide the participant with a basic understanding of healthy leisure. Because the ability to understand a healthy leisure lifestyle is a complex task, Step 3 has six parts. The six parts include the Leisure Level Model, actual participation levels, personal attitudes toward leisure, available leisure time, available resources and leisure interests. In Step 3 the participant gains an awareness of the importance of leisure time and the role that it plays in their life.

The second part of the program relies heavily on "hands on" experiences and encompasses the next three of the eleven steps.

Step 4 is experiential as opposed to cognitive education. The participant experiences leisure participation in the healthy positive levels and receives benefits from each. The participation is clearly led in the direction of health as *no* participation in the unhealthy negative choices is allowed.

Step 5 brings to light unresolved issues of the past and relationship between leisure involvement and what was happening during that time. The participant is able to identify issues such as time frames, related issues and effects on leisure lifestyle, leisure coping mechanisms, social leisure involvement within the time frames, personal feelings associated with past leisure participation, personal leisure choices and leisure barriers. It creates an avenue to assist in sharing with others past issues that may be affecting present and future participation. It is not necessary to be overly specific in what "the past" means, as participants seem able to identify significant issues on their own.

Step 6 deals with planning the future. It assists the participant in identifying the need to structure some aspects of leisure. Without a specific plan many individuals rely totally on spontaneity and rarely follow through with participation on a high leisure level. The plan includes: activity, cost, date, time, with whom, special needs or training and benefits.

The last part of the program consists of the participant actually taking responsibility for his/her own leisure lifestyle, although s/he may still be receiving quite a bit of support from the therapist. The last four steps encourage the participant to "fly on his/her own" under the watchful eye of the therapist. The participant has now participated in assessing needs, setting goals and learning about various aspects of leisure and self. S/he has experienced participating in each (healthy positive) leisure level, explored leisure participation of the past, set a plan for the future and is now ready for participation in all categories of leisure/recreation.

Steps 7,8,9 and 10 involve participating in various categories of leisure activities. Many participants fear participation in the community, as depression, anxiety and other disorders have left the individual unable to handle community level participation. This problem decreases as the participant again becomes familiar with his/her community. This change requires experience, not just verbalization of fears. Without intervention and actual practice the participant many times becomes or remains isolated.

Step 7 gives the participant opportunities to observe leisure activities (Level 1 or Level 2 participation). Being a spectator allows the participant to observe others, allowing less self-consciousness. Many participants express a joy in successful participation. It is a true assessment of the participant's ability of associating with others.

Step 8 includes the leisure areas of arts, crafts, music, drama, dance and home activities. It provides some direction yet allows freedom to choose from the six areas. Many activities from these areas focus on Level 4 participation.

Step 9 includes the leisure areas of exercise, games, sports, physical activities and health. In reading about Step 9 in the instructor's manual the therapist and the participant will easily understand the importance of being active in leading to and maintaining health.

Step 10 is comprised of the areas of education, cultural, volunteerism, collecting and service to others. These areas are many times overlooked by the practitioner as aspects of leisure. Completion of this step has allowed participants to experience choice in all categories of leisure.

An important step, Step 11, offers congratulations to the participant and states to the participant that s/he is free and ready to participate in recreation activities of his/her own choice, time and place and then share the experiences with family, friends and others. This Step takes place after discharge. It offers the participant a review of his/her leisure participation level and compares his/her growth in leisure with Step 3B.

The Mechanics of Running the Program

There are two books that are part of the **Step Up** program. This book contains the instructions for therapist and copies of all of the reproducible sheets for the participant. The second (smaller) book is a workbook for participants in the program. The original purchaser of this book has the licensed right to make as many copies of the workbook as they need for their patients. You may also buy copies of the workbook from Idyll Arbor, if you prefer.

If you choose to make your own copies of the workbook, you should arrange the pages in a three ring binder with dividers separating each step. The participants or staff may complete this task. The therapist may want to use a different colored paper for each step or use standard white paper. With a binder, the participant can take each step from the workbook to work on it and when the step is completed, put it back in the workbook. During treatment, the therapist holds on to the workbook so completed steps don't get lost. Upon discharge, the participant is given his/her accomplishments and instruction for the remaining steps (if there are any). The therapist may take the participant's work out of the three ring binder and place it in a paper notebook, keeping copies of any forms required for documentation.

If you choose to purchase workbooks, be sure to make copies of pages you need for documentation as you go along. This is especially true of the *Step Up Leisure Assessment* in Step 1. The therapist may be creative in how they offer the workbook as a therapeutic intervention.

The therapist will need to compile the resources available in the participant's own community to be able to help the participant through the various steps. Don't just "give" these answers to the participant. One of the most important skills in an independently healthy leisure lifestyle is the ability to go through the phone book, the newspaper or other sources to discover options independently.

The following three pages are the cover and the first two pages of the participant's **Leisure Step Up Workbook**.

Leisure

Step Up

Workbook

Healthy
Choices

Dave Dehn, CTRS

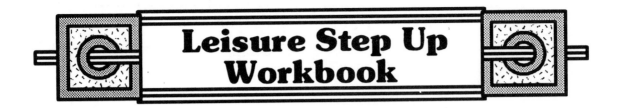

Leisure Step Up Workbook

(Place the name and address of your facility here.
You may also want to include your facility logo.)

Welcome to our program and the **Leisure Step Up Workbook**.
Participation will help you learn positive directions for solving
problems, meeting needs **and** leading a healthy leisure lifestyle.

by Dave Dehn, CTRS, CLP

Idyll Arbor, Inc.

PO Box 720, Ravensdale, WA 98051 (206) 432-3231

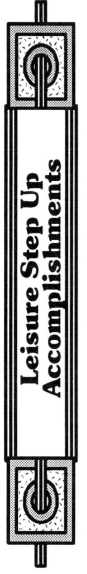

Leisure Step Up Accomplishments

Step Number	Description of Step	Date Accomplished	Staff Initial	Participant Initial	Comments
Step 1	Step Up Leisure Assessment				
Step 2	Leisure Problem Descriptions				
Step 3	Leisure Education Part □ A, □ B, □ C, □ D, □ E, □ F				
Step 4	Recreation Participation				
Step 5	Leisure of the Past				
Step 6	Leisure of the Future				
Step 7	Community Spectator Participation				
Step 8	Expressive Leisure Participation				
Step 9	Physical Leisure Participation				
Step 10	Cultural Leisure Participation				
Step 11	Post - Discharge Recreation Participation				

17

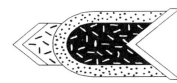 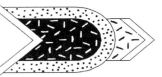

Leisure Level Model

There are two main schools of thought about what "leisure" is. One presents leisure as a state of mind and the other presents leisure as a period of time. The **Leisure Step Up** model combines portions of these two schools of thought. It states that both the degree of emotional and cognitive involvement (state of mind) and the actual participation in leisure activities (time) are important. As with physical and mental health, leisure health is dependent on the participant acting in certain ways (lifestyle) and on the participant thinking in certain ways. To do so requires both continued effort to improve or maintain mental health and also the commitment of time to engage in activities which help maintain or improve one's life.

When you use this book you will be helping the participant understand more about his/her leisure state of mind and use of free time. You will need to measure the participant's current level of involvement with leisure and chart a path to future, healthier levels of leisure.

Participation should be measured as more than attendance at an activity. Participation is a continuum and as such, using a check mark for attendance/participation is relatively meaningless. Nash[2] recognized that participation is a continuum and arranged his leisure continuum much as Maslow arranged his hierarchy of needs. This hierarchy measures leisure participation by how a person uses time for leisure, adding the person's state of mind as one dimension of the hierarchy. Participation — how and why you participate — is something that the participant himself/herself ultimately controls. If the participant is willing to take responsibility for his/her leisure health and is willing to learn how to improve use of leisure time and improve state of mind, s/he will be healthier.

---

[2]Nash, J. B. 1953. **Philosophy of Recreation and Leisure**. Dubuque, Iowa. Wm. C. Brown Company.

Hierarchy of Leisure Participation

Nash first developed a six level model which showed a hierarchy of leisure participation based on the impact of the participation on the individual and those around him/her. His model looked like:

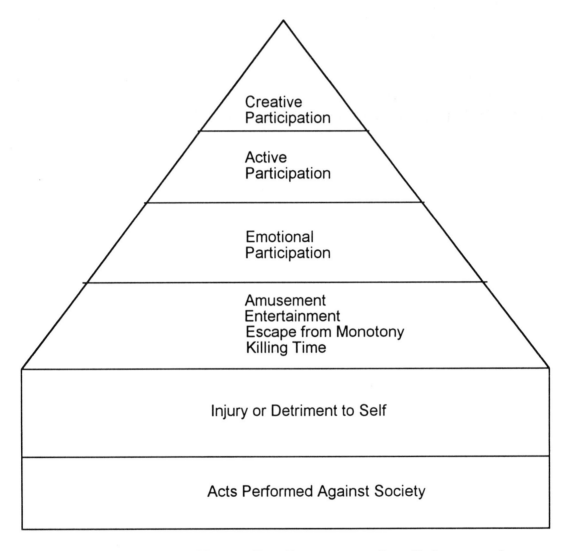

Nash's Model of Man's Use of Leisure Time Participation, Broadly Interpreted.

The most desirable level of participation in Nash's model involved *creative participation*. Those who were creative in their leisure participation tended to be the "makers of the model, the inventor, the painter, the composer". Those who engaged in *active participation* copied the models or played the part that those in the creative participation category developed. Further down on the model was *emotional participation*, those who observed the leisure activities of those who were in the top two levels and were emotionally moved by what they saw. The next level was for those who were not moved by the leisure of others, but who sought out activity to help the *passage of time*. Nash referred to this level as an antidote to boredom.[3]

The last two levels of Nash's models were levels of harm to one's self or to others. The choices made in these levels involved the use of excessive amounts of time in a single or harmful activity or, in the extreme, leisure choices which led to delinquency or crime.

The **Leisure Step Up** program further develops Nash's model into nine levels. These levels emphasize that the participant is at his/her current level as a result of his/her own choices and behaviors. *It is important that the participant develops the awareness that s/he is responsible for his/her leisure.* The therapist must feel that s/he has a solid understanding of the leisure model before s/he can successfully help the participant move through all eleven steps of the program.

For the participant to make good, purposeful choices about his/her leisure, s/he needs to know the breadth of choices between very unhealthy leisure activity and very healthy, cathartic leisure activity. Teaching the participant about his/her choices using the Leisure Level Model (See the chart on the following page.) is the basic foundation for the **Leisure Step Up** program.

---

[3]We now know that there are two different causes for boredom. In addition to a lack of things to do, boredom may also be the person's response to over stimulation or more choices then s/he can handle. The body has literally "shut down" because of the inability to control the amount and quality of stimuli and choices. If a person is participating at this level, it may mean that the therapist will need to help structure the environment so that it is producing less stimuli and offering fewer choices before the patient can physiologically reach a level of stability to be able to make choices which more actively engage him/her during leisure time.

21

Leisure Level Model

The activities that I choose to participate in during my free time.

⟹	**Healthy Positive Choices**	

	Cathartic Level

My Choices/My Behavior. My participation reaches a point of catharsis. My participation makes a measurable change in my life. **Examples:** vacation, climbing a mountain, prayer, ropes course, watching an event, achieving the goal, etc.

⟹	**Level 4**

My Choices/My Behavior. I am creative, inventive, imaginative, taking nothing and making something. Not following a plan or instruction. **Examples:** Poetry, drawing, painting, crafts, cooking, sculpting, music, prayer, etc.

⟹	**Level 3**

My Choices/My Behavior. I am active physically, socially and/or cognitively. Activity follows instruction, a plan, rules, with participation on an emotional level. **Examples:** Crafts, cooking, bike riding, sports participation, intense laughter (internal jogging), dancing, games, skateboarding, reading, physical workout, relaxation therapy, etc.

⟹	**Level 2**

My Choices/My Behavior. I am a spectator emotionally involved. There is a personal investment, true entertainment. **Examples:** TV, radio, watching others participate in Level 3 and 4 activities.

⟹	**Level 1**

My Choices/My Behavior. I am a spectator with no emotional involvement. Participation lacks personal investment, *positive* activities with nothing else to do. **Examples:** Watching TV, listening to the radio, watching others participate in Level 3 and 4 activities.

⟸	**Level 0**

My Choices/My Behavior. Participation could be forced, obligated, duty, with no internalization of participation. Preoccupation during participation in Level 1, 2, 3 or 4 activities. **Examples:**

⟸	**Unhealthy Negative Choices**	**Level -1**

My Choices/My Behavior. I am preoccupied in thought or feeling and just going through the motions of the activity. Participation could be forced, obligated, duty, with no internalization of participation. **Examples:**

My Choices/My Behavior. I am harmed physically, mentally or emotionally. **Examples:** Substance abuse, dangerous high risk activities, self abuse, negative thinking, poor dietary choices, too much or not enough sleeping, eating, exercising, relaxing, etc.

⟸	**Level -2**

My Choices/My Behavior. I affect others in a harmful or hurting manner. This includes physical, emotional or mental harm to my family, friends or community. **Examples:** Substance abuse, inappropriate competition, gossip, threatening, name calling, fighting, hurting animals, breaking the law (minor), no family time, etc.

⟸	**Lost Freedom**

My Choices/My Behavior. I harm myself or others. My behavior causes a loss in freedom to choose my own leisure. Often the victim's and/or family's leisure are also affected. **Examples:** Crime, gang involvement, vandalism, fighting, suicide gestures, breaking the law (major: rape, self abuse, sexual abuse, substance abuse, etc.).

Unhealthy Leisure Participation Levels

The very bottom of the model reflects a state of *lost freedom* and choices in leisure activity because of previous, unhealthy and/or illegal activity on the part of the participant. The next two levels, both still considered to be unhealthy, reflect leisure choices made by the participant which have either harmed others (*Level -2*) or harmed himself/herself (*Level -1*). If the participant remains at any of these three levels, it is unlikely that s/he will be able to obtain an overall "healthy" status — in leisure or otherwise. To be able to achieve greater health, the participant will need to choose to make purposeful change (and then make that change) in his/her leisure activity to be able to move toward greater health.

Lost Freedom often involves the voluntary or involuntary commitment to an institution. The participant's behavior has been so unacceptable that it caused a loss of freedom to choose his/her own leisure. Some examples are crime, gang involvement, vandalism, fighting, suicide gestures, breaking the law (major violations such as rape, sexual abuse, substance abuse). As a result of the participant's previous actions, others have imposed severe limits on his/her leisure choices. A state of mind can also cause lost freedom, perhaps an even more serious loss than confinement in an institution. One example is a rape victim who loses freedom to choose leisure activities because of fear, guilt and/or depression. Another example might be a person who has lost a close family member and cannot make leisure choices because of anger, depression or mourning. Most participants who are at this level are in significant need of learning new leisure patterns. Counseling is often necessary for the participant to return to healthy choices.

Level -2 frequently involves some limitation on the participant's leisure as a direct result of his/her previous actions. The participant's choices and behavior has affected others in a harmful or hurting manner. This behavior may have included such things as physical, emotional or mental harm to his/her family, friends, others or the community. Some examples would be substance abuse, inappropriate competition, gossip, threatening others, name calling, fighting, hurting animals, breaking the law (minor offenses), deserting or ignoring family, etc. The degree to which his/her leisure is controlled by others may not be as significant as in the Lost Freedom Level, but, because it has led to the harm of others, society has placed some limits on his/her freedom. Participants in this level may need to concentrate on learning good, basic social skills (and respect) on a one to one basis or in small groups first. Often on this level denial is a mask. The participant may believe that s/he is having fun and meeting his/her needs. In actuality needs are not being met and the participant may be spiraling down toward lost freedom.

Level -1 involves the participation in leisure activities that are harmful to him/herself, but which may not be the primary reason for admission to a treatment program. The participant's choices and behavior affects himself/herself, his/her health and welfare so that s/he is harmed physically, mentally or emotionally. Some examples of activities which would place the participant in this level would be substance abuse, dangerous high risk

23

activities,[4] self abuse, negative thinking, poor dietary choices, too much or not enough sleeping, eating, exercising, relaxing, etc.

Neutral Leisure Participation

Level "0" (zero) is a neutral-to-negative position related to leisure activity. The participant tends to be preoccupied in thought or feeling and s/he is just going through the motions of the activity. If the participant is engaging in activities that would normally be a higher level but remains preoccupied through the activity, s/he is functioning at Level 0. Usually this level results when the participant has such a high level of stress, frustration, depression, etc. that s/he spends much more energy worrying about his/her problems than about the activity s/he is participating in. If a participant chooses to participate in his/her leisure activities at this level s/he will have a difficult time reaching true health. However, if Level 0 is a step or two above where s/he was before, participation at this level could be an encouraging sign.

Healthy Leisure Participation Levels

On the Leisure Level Model, Levels 1, 2, 3, 4 and the Cathartic Level are all healthy levels of leisure participation. The participant may be involved at numerous levels. With increased awareness and skill, all the levels of healthy leisure will be available to the participant.

Level 1 involves a minimal amount of healthy leisure. The participant's choices and behaviors are those of a spectator without any emotional involvement in the activity. The participant tends to lack personal investment in positive leisure activities, with little to fill his/her time. Examples of activities which tend to support this kind of participation are watching television, listening to the radio or watching others participate in the more positive levels of leisure.

Level 2 requires little active participation in leisure activities but does have the healthy attribute of having the participant emotionally involved in what s/he is observing. The participant's choices and behaviors indicate a personal investment in the activity, an interest which, in turn, allows the observed leisure activity to be entertaining. Examples of activities which tend to support this kind of participation include watching sports and watching others participate in higher level activities.

Level 3 participation is an upper level in the Leisure Level Model continuum. When defining recreation most people think of activity on this level. At this level the participant

---

[4]High risk activities do not automatically mean that the patient should be placed at this level. High risk activities are activities which require instruction, lengthy training and practice to be able to perform safely. If the patient engages in high risk activities without the proper training, instruction, and practice, then the patient's participation in the activity should be considered to be dangerous.

is a player as opposed to a spectator as in Levels 1 and 2. It includes cognitive, physical and/or social parts. All of these parts are important. One is not a substitute for the other, as we must participate in some element of physical, social and cognitive activity on a regular basis to be healthy. A key point in this level is following a plan, instruction or rules during participation.

The physical category is extremely important in therapy and needs to be a part of every participant's life to help maintain health. Physical activity and exercise may be the most used and highly accepted therapeutic programming approach in recreational therapy. The recreational therapist must use caution in programming because participants with mental or chemical dependency problems will often be in poor physical condition. Examples of physical participation include: riding a bike, fly fishing, weight training, walking a nature trail, following an instructor in aerobic exercise, playing racquetball, jogging or dancing the fox-trot.

The cognitive category includes the thinking process. Cognitive aspects are important because many participants with mental health issues may not be thinking clearly, while many participants with chemical dependencies suffer from brain damage. Participation in cognitive activities sharpens thought process leading to improved decision making, listening skills, improved memory, etc. Examples of cognitive participation are reading a "how to repair" book; playing a game of strategy, chess, clue, memory; reminiscing while watching home movies; working on puzzles, math problems, word problems; or following instructions in building a model ship.

The social category includes verbal and/or non-verbal conversation/interaction with at least one other person. Participation must include emotional involvement or the socialization would be on a lower level. Usually participants think social activities include sitting down with a friend and carrying on a conversation or being at a party or engagement with a group. While this is true, socialization also includes non-verbal participation in recreation activities. The action, the play, the movement are the means of communication. Examples include playing checkers, basketball, table games, sport activity and group projects.

It is not necessarily important to decide if an activity is physical, social or cognitive. The decision however would be which aspects are considered important during participation. For a healthy leisure the participant needs to have some of each. How s/he mixes and matches activities to get all three aspects is an important aspect of the therapeutic process.

Level 4 participation offers a means of expressing emotions. It is above Level 3 in emotive expression, in that participation does not follow a plan, patterns or instruction. The participants leave part of themselves in what they accomplish and what they accomplish becomes part of them. Many poets, artists and musicians describe this level of participation as including their soul, the essence of their existence. A key phrase is taking nothing and making something. Examples are taking a lump of clay and molding a figure, writing a short story, cooking from scratch (no recipe), talking to God from your heart, making plans to decorate for a party or unstructured free play.

Contrary to what the participant may believe, this level can be achieved by learning and practicing. Some people say, "I'm not a creative person." However, creativity can be learned. Just like all good things, it takes work (or play, depending on the perception of leisure) to be successfully creative. As a therapist you can help each participant find his/her natural creativity and help it grow.

Cathartic Level is the ultimate level in leisure participation. It is free time participation that is extremely emotional. When a participant is participating in Level 2, 3 or 4 activities, s/he may reach a cathartic point. Many times that feeling of personal growth acts as a catalyst for a change in the participant's lifestyle. You cannot plan to achieve this level. It happens as a result of the right chemistry of emotional state and the activity. It is participation on a Level 2, 3 or 4 that has a lasting and memorable effect on the participant. Examples are watching a movie that portrays an aspect of the individual's life and teaches a value, talking to God and gaining inspiration, going on a family vacation that solidifies family ties.

Summary: The Leisure Level Model is a tool that gives value to choices and behaviors during leisure time. It can help the participant see that what s/he does with his/her leisure time does make a difference. It gives participants a goal to achieve. The participants do not always need to participate on a high level. They need to find a balance among the positive Levels 1 through 4, while staying away from participation on the negative levels.

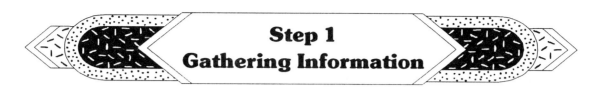

Step 1
Gathering Information

The **Leisure Step Up** program begins with an assessment of the current functional level of the participant. The **Leisure Step Up** initial assessment tools consist of a portion the participant fills out and the GALF Scale scored by the therapist from information about the participant. In addition to the assessment, there is an information sheet that the therapist may use to gather more information about the participant if it is not available in the participant's chart. For most participants the information gathered by these tools will be enough to develop treatment objectives.

However, no one testing tool will provide the therapist with what s/he needs to know about every participant prior to providing treatment. Some participants will be admitted who have specialized needs. In those cases, the therapist may want to use additional testing tools to supplement or replace the **Leisure Step Up** tools. While the majority of participants will only need the assessment tools contained in this book, we have included suggestions about other testing tools in the section on *Treatment Directions in Leisure* which may help the therapist make sounder clinical decisions.

The following is an outline of what you do for Step 1.

1. Study the background information of the participant before the Step Up Leisure Assessment. Often a social history, medical history, intake interview, physical exam, staffing report and previous admission information will be available in the participant's chart.
2. If necessary, arrange a time for observing the participant and conducting the assessment and interview.
3. Give the participant a brief explanation and directions for the Step Up Leisure Assessment. Have the participant fill out the Step Up Leisure Assessment. The Step Up Information Handout (at the end of Step 1) may also be given at this time. It is a quick reference which can be used during the interview or for setting therapeutic goals and behavioral objectives. The therapist need not be present at this time if the participant does not need assistance.
4. Interview the participant regarding the assessment. Focus on low functioning areas, gaining specific functional information on the participant's attitude, thoughts, feelings and, most important, information on the participant's behaviors. Information on high functioning areas can be helpful for programming purposes and knowing the participant's strengths. The interview takes approximately 15 minutes unless the participant needs further assistance or counseling.
5. Assess the Domains by taking the low functioning scores of the domain and applying them to the Leisure Assessment scoring key. Fill in the score and level.
6. Assess the Global Assessment Leisure Functioning (GALF) by taking functional information, observations and other information to determine a GALF score.

27

7. Write a brief explanation of significant functional information, the participant's recreational therapy treatment goals and behavioral objectives. The goals and objectives may be changed as needed and new treatment goals or objectives may be set as needs are met and problems are solved. The Step Up Leisure Assessment, participant interview and write up will usually take approximately 30 minutes.

Background Information

Prior to administering the assessments in the **Leisure Step Up**, the therapist should review information found in the participant's chart. This review is done for three reasons:

1. to familiarize the therapist with the reason(s) for admission and anticipated discharge date,
2. to develop an understanding of the participant's social, educational, vocational and economic background and
3. to note information about safety concerns and medications.

The information found in the medical chart will guide the therapist as s/he starts to formulate a treatment intervention.

Leisure Step Up Initial Assessment

The **Leisure Step Up** Initial Assessment consists of two parts: the Step Up Leisure Assessment and the Global Assessment and Leisure Functioning (GALF) Scale.

The Step Up Leisure Assessment is given to the participant who should complete it as independently as possible. It takes most participants on a psychiatric unit 15-30 minutes to complete.

The second tool, the GALF Scale, is completed by the recreational therapist after:
1. reviewing the participant's chart
2. conducting an interview with the participant
3. scoring the Step Up Leisure Assessment.

The Step Up Leisure Assessment is an initial, baseline assessment. The assessment has been developed for age thirteen years or above, with an IQ at eighty or above. It is divided into six domains: Leisure Functioning, Physical Functioning, Cognitive Functioning, Daily Living Functioning, Social Functioning and Psychological Functioning. The domains may be addressed separately or as a global assessment. Each domain covers an important aspect of recreational therapy.

The assessment is designed to gather as much information about the participant as possible. When the therapist analyzes the answers, s/he needs to remember that the answers are coming from a participant perspective and may need to be substantiated through participant interview, observation, social history and other various forms of documentation and resources. The questions 1, 2, 3, 5 and 6 of each domain score lower functioning for a lower number. Questions 4 and 7 score lower functioning for a higher number. This helps identify participants that do not understand or are not reading each question carefully. The questions are presented in a format that is easy to understand. However, it may be necessary to read or have someone read the questions if the participant's reading or visual skills are inadequate. The Step Up Leisure Assessment has a Flesch Grade Level of 6.8.

The answers are coded with the numbers 1, 2, 3, 4 and 5 which mean almost never, rarely, sometimes, usually and almost always. The numbers help the therapist in scoring while the terms help the participant's understanding of the answers.

The therapist need not be present while the participant fills out the assessment after a brief and clear explanation of the screening tool. However, a participant interview is essential in case the participant has questions or to further explore low and high functioning scores. Exploration of the deficits and/or strengths usually takes 15–20 minutes, however, the therapist must be sensitive to the participant's needs and allow more time in scheduling if necessary.

Give the Leisure Assessment sheet shown on the next page to the participant and tell him/her:

> **Please read each question carefully, being honest with each question. After you read each sentence, you are asked to indicate how much that sentence describes how you feel. "1" means almost never, "2" means rarely, "3" means sometimes, "4" means usually and "5" means almost always.**

When the participant is finished, take the completed form and score it. In the meantime you will usually let the participant fill out the information handout.

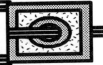

Step 1
Leisure Assessment

Directions: Please read each question carefully, being honest with each question. After you read each sentence, indicate how much that sentence describes how you feel using the scale below.

1. Almost Never	2. Rarely	3. Sometimes	4. Usually	5. Almost Always

Leisure Functioning

___ 1. The things I do with my free time are positive.

___ 2. I get to do the things I want to with my free time.

___ 3. I enjoy my free time.

___ 4. When I get free time, I do not know what to do.

___ 5. I get enough free time.

___ 6. I am interested in learning new things to do.

___ 7. My free time is boring.

Physical Functioning

___ 1. I like the way I look.

___ 2. I am physically active.

___ 3. I feel good physically.

___ 4. My physical health and condition prevent me from doing what I want.

___ 5. I get enough sleep.

___ 6. I have enough energy.

___ 7. My drug or alcohol use creates problems.

Cognitive Functioning

___ 1. I can concentrate or focus on a task.

___ 2. I can participate in the same activity for a long period of time.

___ 3. I can think clearly in solving my problems.

___ 4. I forget things that happened to me and what I did when I was young.

___ 5. I know where I am, what day it is and what I am doing.

___ 6. I understand directions or rules.

___ 7. Ten minutes after I see, read or hear something I forget what it was.

Daily Living Functioning

___ 1. I feel safe in my home.

___ 2. I eat a balanced diet.

___ 3. I bathe or shower daily and take care of my health.

___ 4. I have problems with those I work or go to school with.

___ 5. I attend my school or job.

___ 6. I participate in cleaning, cooking and responsibilities at home.

___ 7. I have problems with school/job or my daily responsibilities.

Social Functioning

___ 1. I share my feelings.

___ 2. I can depend upon my friends.

___ 3. I get along with authority.

___ 4. I avoid time alone.

___ 5. My family is important to me.

___ 6. I enjoy being around others.

___ 7. I give in to peer pressure.

Psychological Functioning

___ 1. I think positively about myself.

___ 2. My stress level is manageable.

___ 3. I make good decisions.

___ 4. I feel depressed.

___ 5. I am calm and in control.

___ 6. I behave in a rational manner.

___ 7. My attitude leads to problems.

30

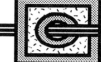

Step 1
Assessment Summary

Functional Ability:

Leisure Functioning: _____

Physical Functioning: _____

Cognitive Functioning: _____

Daily Living Functioning: _____

Social Functioning: _____

Psychological Functioning: _____

Global Assessment and Leisure Functioning (GALF) SCALE: _____

Comments/Summary:

Treatment Goals and Objectives:

Participant _____ **Date** _____ **Staff** _____

Step Up Assessment Summary

The Step Up Assessment Summary shown on the previous page has areas for scoring the Step Up Leisure Assessment, for entering a Global Assessment and Leisure Functioning Scale level, for writing additional comments and observations and for documenting the initial treatment goals and objectives.

It is essential to include the Step Up Leisure Assessment in the participant's permanent record. You may modify the summary sheet as required to meet the documentation standards of your facility.

Step Up Leisure Assessment Scoring

Assessment screen areas include: Leisure Functioning, Physical Functioning, Cognitive Functioning, Daily Living Functioning, Social Functioning and Psychological Functioning.

There is a score for each question. The lowest level of functioning in each domain dictates the level of functioning in that domain. The more impairment/deficiency scores the person has within the domain, the greater the area of dysfunction. The high functioning scores can be used as a strength in programming to assist in problem solving.

In questions 1, 2, 3, 5 and 6: *almost never* (1) is the lowest functioning level and *almost always* (5) is the highest. In questions 4 and 7: *almost never* (1) is the highest functioning level and *almost always* (5) is the lowest.

Each question is assessed separately and then the scores are combined for an overall domain score. For example, the chart below shows scores in the Leisure Functioning Domain with the scores you would assign:

question	participant's answer	your score for the answer
1	2	low functioning
2	5	high functioning
3	5	high functioning
4	4	low functioning (questions 4 and 7 are reversed)
5	5	high functioning
6	2	low functioning
7	1	high functioning (questions 4 and 7 are reversed)

Scoring for the whole domain goes as follows:

If the participant reports:	The domain represents:
High functioning (All scores of 1 or 5)	Strength
Average functioning (All scores at least 2 or 4)	Acceptable
Below Average (Any one score of 3)	Mild impairment
Low Functioning (Any one score of 2 or 4)	Moderate impairment
Low Functioning (Any one score of 1 or 5)	Deficit

In the example of the Leisure Functioning Domain shown above, the participant would have a score of <u>low functioning x 3 deficit</u> from questions 1, 4 and 6.

Global Assessment and Leisure Functioning (GALF) Scale Scoring

The GALF Scale is a single rating scale that is used for evaluating functional levels in the areas of leisure, education, psychological functioning, social interactions, daily living (including home, occupation, school), physical abilities and cognition.

The GALF scale was devised by adding Leisure aspects to the Global Assessment and Functioning Scale (GAF scale) taken from Axis IV, Diagnostic Criteria from DSM-IV[5].

In rating a person, information can be taken from the Leisure Assessment, participant interview, participant documentation, observation, other staff and other reliable sources. Like the (GAF), ratings can be made for two time periods.
1. Functional level at the time of the assessment.
2. Functional levels during the past year (high and/or low)

Functional level at the time of the assessment will assist in setting a participant treatment plan and in therapeutic programming. Functional levels of the past year will help the therapist gain knowledge of the participant's enduring strengths and weaknesses. This will also be helpful in monitoring outcomes and in long range goal setting. The scale ranges from 1–100, from unhealthy to healthy.

The scale is divided into ten intervals. Functional levels can be determined within a level by assessing if the functional level is closer to the level above or below e.g., a person unable to keep a job would be functioning on the scale from 50–41. However, there is difficulty associated with the person receiving pleasure from leisure involvement. The therapist would then subjectively decide that the person falls into the lower part of the range for a score of 41, 42 or 43.

---

[5]The GALF scale is a revision of the GAF scale, from the American Psychiatric Association, 1994, **American Psychiatric Association: Diagnostic and Statistical Manual of Mental Health Disorders, Fourth Edition**. Washington, DC. Used with permission.

When entering the score on the Step Up Assessment Summary, be sure to enter both the number and a brief description of the meaning of the number so that other team members who are not familiar with the scale will be able to understand your evaluation. (For example, 66 – mild symptoms of dysfunction.)

A person's current functional level is determined by the lowest point of functioning. Functional levels (high and low) during the past year should include at least a three month period, part of which should include a time period of school or work.

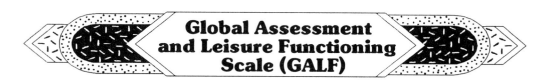

Global Assessment and Leisure Functioning Scale (GALF)

100 91	Superior functioning in a wide range of activities, life's problems never seem to get out of hand, is sought out by others because of his/her many positive qualities. Well balanced leisure lifestyle. No problems.
90 81	Absent or minimal symptoms (e.g., mild anxiety before an exam), good functioning in all areas, has knowledge, skills, interest and involved in a wide range of activities, (e.g., initiates positive leisure involvement), socially effective, an ability to share/express feelings, generally satisfied with life, no more than everyday problems or concerns (e.g., an occasional argument with family members).
80 71	If symptoms are present, they are transient and expectable reactions to psychosocial stresses (e.g., difficulty concentrating after family argument), no more than slight impairment in leisure, occupational or school functioning (e.g., temporarily falling behind in schoolwork, postponement of leisure plans, temporary increase in caffeine, junk food or smoking).
70 61	Some mild symptoms (e.g., depressed mood, lack of motivation or energy, mild insomnia) or some difficulty in leisure, occupational or school functioning (e.g., occasional threats or theft within the household, occasionally involved in altercations with peers, coming home late beyond curfew), but generally functioning pretty well, has some meaningful interpersonal relationships, some structure to components of leisure time, (e.g., member of a club or organization of a positive nature).
60 51	Moderate symptoms (e.g., flat affect and circumstantial speech, occasional panic attacks) or moderate difficulty in leisure, occupational, school functioning (e.g., few friends, conflicts with co-workers, loss of interest in recreational activities, pre-occupation during leisure time).
50 41	Serious symptoms (e.g., suicidal ideation, severe obsessional rituals, frequent shoplifting) or any serious impairment in leisure, occupational or school functioning (e.g., no friends, unable to keep a job, recreational choices determined by substance abuse, unkempt personal hygiene, extremely short attention span, frequent conflict with authority figures, fear of recreation within the community).
40 31	Some impairment in reality testing or communication (e.g., speech is at times illogical, obscure or irrelevant) or major impairment in several areas such as work, school, leisure, family relations, judgment, thinking or mood (e.g., man who is depressed avoids friends, neglects family and is unable to work; child who frequently beats up younger children, is defiant at home, is failing school, lacks ability to concentrate or follow process of play/games, fears being alone, sporadic eating or frequent purging, no energy or interest, inability to receive pleasure from pleasurable activities).
30 21	Behavior is considerably influenced by delusions or hallucinations or serious impairment in communication or judgment (e.g., sometimes incoherent, acts grossly inappropriately, suicidal preoccupation) or inability to function in almost all areas (e.g., stays in bed all day, no job, home, friends, play or recreation).
20 11	Some danger of hurting self or others (e.g., suicide attempts without clear expectation of death, frequently violent, manic excitement), participates in frequent dangerous leisure activities with little thought of consequences, (e.g., playing chicken with a moving vehicle, cliff diving with no precautions, almost always intoxicated) or occasionally fails to maintain minimal personal hygiene (e.g., smears feces) or gross impairment in communication (e.g., largely incoherent or mute, frequent abuse/neglect of children).
10 1	Persistent danger of severely hurting self or others (e.g., recurrent violence, violent daily gang activity) or persistent inability to maintain minimal personal hygiene or serious suicidal act with clear expectation of death (e.g., recurrent drug overdose).

Modified, with permission, from the GAF, American Psychiatric Association, 1994

Comments/Summary

The Comments/Summary section should include specific information from the assessment interview about the participant's current leisure activities, both positive and negative. Other personal, family, school or work information that is relevant to the treatment plan should also be included. For example:

This participant is not engaged in positive activity during leisure time, i.e. constant sibling conflict and stealing from stores. She is lacking in interest in leisure activity and has no knowledge of home or community resources. Note that the participant has recently moved from Denver to live with her mother in this community.

Written Treatment Plan

A written treatment plan consisting of Participant Goals and Objectives should address deficits found in the Step Up Leisure Assessment. A written treatment plan is essential in giving treatment direction and in monitoring participant progress toward the desired outcome.

Goals are made up of three components:
1) problem
2) need in relation to problem
3) goal in relation to need

Example 1:
Problem: constant sibling conflict with physical altercations
Need: to stop physical altercations and reduce conflict
Goal: no physical altercations with sibling and conflict brought down to a minimum

Example 2:
Problem: stealing from community stores
Need: to completely stop stealing
Goal: no stealing behaviors

Objectives put the goal statement into behavioral terms. There are three components of a behavioral objective:
1) specific behaviors
2) conditions (where and when)
3) measurable standards (how much, how often)

It is extremely important for each objective to be easily measured so that both the therapist and the participant can tell how closely the behaviors match the objectives.

Example 1:
Behavior: Participant will interact in conversation in a social manner ...
Conditions: when in the same room with her siblings ...
Standards: at least half of the time during the next three weeks.

Example 2:
Behavior: There will be no more instances of stealing ...
Conditions: at any time ...
Standards: starting immediately.

Complete Behavioral Objectives

Example 1:
The participant will list 10 community resources this Friday in leisure education group therapy, choosing one to attend while on weekend pass.

Example 2:
*The participant will demonstrate a decrease in anger by **no** physical threats, after two weeks of recreational therapy exercise groups 3 times a week and completion of an anger management course.*

Step Up Recreational Therapy Information Handout

The Step Up Recreational Therapy Information Handout should be given to each participant during Step 1. It allows the participant to talk about his/her perception of important elements in his/her life. The therapist should already know some of the information from researching the participant's history so the form can also be used as a measure of how well the participant understands his/her own situation.

Have the participant fill in the form as independently as possible and go over the answers at the same time you discuss the other information gathered during Step 1.

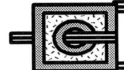

Step 1
Information Handout

Name _____   **Date** _____

Directions: Please fill in the blank spaces provided.

My main reason for coming in for treatment is _____

_____

_____

Things I do with my free time include:

_____   _____

_____   _____

Things that prevent me from doing what I want are

_____   _____

_____   _____

List any physical/health problems or allergies:

_____   _____

_____   _____

I am employed or have been employed in the past: ☐ No ☐ Yes
If Yes, ☐ Past ☐ Currently

My job was/is _____ I work(ed) _____ hours per week

If I had any problems with my job, it was _____

_____

I currently attend school: ☐ No ☐ Yes
If Yes, I am in the _____ grade.
My average grades are _____.

My relationships with teachers are
☐ pleasant   ☐ friendly   ☐ so-so   ☐ unfriendly   ☐ disgusting

Explain: _____

_____

My relationships with peers are _____

_____

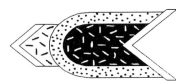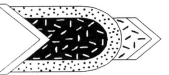

Step 2
Leisure Plan

Step 2 involves creating a leisure plan for and with the participant. This plan includes specific leisure goals that the participant will aim to accomplish throughout the rest of the **Leisure Step Up** program. Included in this step are a set of problem areas and programmatic ideas. The Leisure Plan information may also be helpful in revising the participant's treatment plan written in Step 1.

The participant's success in the Leisure Plan is more likely to take place if the participant:

1. Has a clear understanding of the directions.
2. Believes that leisure participation is therapeutic and problem solving.
3. Is motivated or will become increasingly motivated with participation in the plan.
4. Plays a part is setting the Leisure Plan.
5. Understands the plan because it is simple and attainable.

The Leisure Plan should be flexible, as further participation in the **Leisure Step Up** program will help the participant change attitude, develop skills and increase awareness of self and leisure. Thus the plan may be changed, completed or added to as required by the participant's current treatment needs.

Individualizing a participant's treatment is extremely important in offering a good quality, therapeutic program. The therapy should be tailored to the individual by setting individual goals, counseling in specific skills and working throughout the process to meet each participant's personal requirements.

It is important to work closely with other health care professionals to create a cohesive overall treatment plan. In this way, the participant will be given various methodologies and means of dealing with his/her problems. Examples of this are educational groups, family therapy, cognitive groups, occupational therapy, psychotherapy, recreational therapy, music therapy, art therapy, dance therapy, etc. Each of these deals with the participant's various problems from different perspectives, offering many frameworks as a therapeutic approach.

The Leisure Plan portion of Step 2 has two parts: a page for the problem description and a page for the corresponding solutions.

Leisure Plan Part A: Problem Descriptions

This part consists of writing problems and a brief description of the problem. Many participants will need only minimal assistance, if any, in completing Part A. Many problems will coincide with the participant's treatment plan. However, these will be in the participant's words and from his/her perspective. Some participants may forget, neglect or deny certain problems that need to be addressed during the participant's treatment. Identification of a problem is the first step in problem solving and it is up to the therapist to see that the participant identifies at least some of the significant problems in this step.

Examples of Problems and Descriptions:

Problem	Brief Description
Anger, out of control	I am extremely angry over my past sexual abuse, I get mad and blow up at anything.
I don't know what to do with my time, I'm depressed	I watch TV or sleep most of the day. I don't have any friends. I have used drugs and alcohol in the past.
I constantly fight with my family especially my mom.	My mom and I constantly fight. She never lets me do anything with my friends, so I sneak out anyway. I don't trust her.

Leisure Plan Part B: Problem Solutions

Part B individualizes the participant's leisure direction and includes them in planning the treatment. They may need a lot of assistance in applying leisure participation to problem solving. The Leisure Plan may coincide with the participant's treatment plan, in goal setting or behavioral objectives, but it is best if it is written in the participant's own words.

Examples of a Leisure Plan

Problem	Leisure Plan
Anger, out of control	Attend anger reduction group on Tuesdays, practice relaxation technique. When I feel I'm getting angry, I will use the relaxation techniques I learned.
Don't know what to do with my leisure time, I'm depressed.	Complete Step 3 of **Leisure Step Up** by August 10th, participate in a positive healthy leisure activity for one hour a day instead of sleeping or watching TV, read article on "making friends".
I constantly fight with my family, especially my mom.	Participate in family night activities with my family (no fighting), on weekend passes, help my mom with the chores, clean bathrooms, vacuum, do the dishes, etc. Also on pass go bowling with the family, have a heart to heart talk with mom during visiting hour.

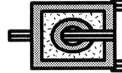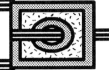

Step 2 Part A
Problem Descriptions

Name _____   **Date** _____

Directions: List three major problems and write a brief description of each problem.

1. Problem:

    Description:

2. Problem:

    Description:

3. Problem:

    Description:

4. Other problem areas include:

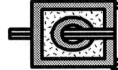 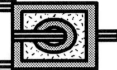

Step 2 Part B
Problem Solutions

Name _____   **Date** _____

Directions: With the help of the recreational therapist, write down recreation and leisure goals which will help solve the problems you listed.

1. Problem:

   Leisure Goal:

2. Problem:

   Leisure Goal:

3. Problem:

   Leisure Goal:

4. Other goals include:

Functional Disorders and Treatment Directions

If you or the participant are having trouble identifying problems, the next page shows a list of problems which are often associated with deficits identified in Step 1. The pages following that show goals and treatment directions (ways of accomplishing the goal) for each problem described in the problem list. Of course, the list is not complete, so as you identify new problems, goals or pathways, you can add them to the following pages.

There are countless activity books, game books, leisure books, etc. from many professions that can be used to add to the Leisure Plan column. The more resources available to the therapist the greater chance of meeting each participant's needs. To increase the Leisure Plan list for a particular problem, the therapist must look at the benefit and the outcome for the particular activity. If the result of the activity meets the participant's goals, participation in that activity will help the participant improve functionality within the particular domain.

The Leisure Plan, as you can see from the following pages can be drawn from six domains: Leisure Functioning, Physical Functioning, Cognitive Functioning, Daily Living Functioning, Social Functioning and Psychological Functioning. The problems are listed under a particular domain. Many problems could be in several functional domains. An example of this would be an eating disorder problem. This problem could be under the domain of Physical Functioning as well as Daily Living Functioning.

The domains are all connected. It is very important to consider the total person in treatment and not just one aspect or domain. Low functioning in any domain will affect all domains in some respect and will affect that mental health of the individual. The old adage of treating the person and not the problem remains important in quality treatment. Another concept of equal importance is that the approach and manner that you use to deliver the Leisure Plan is of more importance than prescribing the exact correct activity. (It's not what you do, it's how you do it.) The therapist should help the participant pick problems and goals that will make a significant difference in his/her life.

Functional Disorders Impacting Leisure Performance

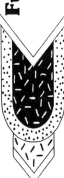

LEISURE FUNCTIONING	PHYSICAL FUNCTIONING	COGNITIVE FUNCTIONING	DAILY LIVING	SOCIAL FUNCTIONING	PSYCHOLOGICAL FUNCTIONING
Lack of leisure or free time awareness	Lack of motivation, energy (lethargic)	Lack of problem solving skills	Unsafe living environment	Peer or authority conflicts	Pre-occupation with problem
Lack of leisure skills	Inappropriate somatic complaints	Attention deficit	Poor personal health or hygiene	Family conflict, parent/child conflict	Fear of failure, success
Lack of knowledge of home or community leisure resources	Insomnia	Poor decision making skills	Poor living skills (cooking, cleaning, house-hold tasks)	Lack of support systems	Unmanageable stress/anxiety/panic attacks
Anhedonic (unable to receive pleasure from pleasurable activities)	Substance Abuse	Lack of recollection, memory	Lack of success with school or employment	Lack of trust	Lack of ability to express feelings
Lack of positive healthy leisure coping mechanisms	Eating disorders: Obesity, Anorexia, Bulimia	Obsessive thoughts, compulsive behavior		Lack of communication skills	Inappropriate affect
Excessive use of leisure or workaholic				Social isolation	Delusions or hallucinations
Lack of leisure interests					Low self esteem
					Oppositional defiant behaviors/conduct disorders
					Out of control anger/rage

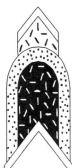

Treatment Directions In Leisure

Leisure Functioning Domain

Problem	Goal	Treatment Directions
Lack of leisure or free time awareness	Increase leisure or free time awareness	**Determining Functional Level** • Idyll Arbor Leisure Battery — Leisure Attitude Measurement, Leisure Interest Measurement, Leisure Motivation Scale, Leisure Satisfaction Measure (Beard and Ragheb, 1989) • Step 3 of Leisure Step Up • STILAP (Navar, 1990) • Leisure Diagnostic Battery (Witt and Ellis, 1982) **Treatment Directions** The general concern for the therapist in this situation is to: 1. determine if the participant is oriented enough to understand the concept that s/he is responsible for his/her leisure time, 2. assist the participant in developing an awareness of his/her leisure time, 3. assist the participant in the process of appropriately reclaiming some time for positive leisure experiences and 4. help the participant gain understanding about using leisure to improve and maintain his/her health.
Lack of leisure skills	Increase leisure skills in various areas	**Determining Functional Level** • Assessment in leisure skills (skiing, bowling, hiking, biking, pottery, sewing, swimming, cooking) using such tools as the ICAN Program (Wessel, 1979), material from the American Red Cross • Leisure Step Up Steps 8, 9, 10 (golf, skating, yoga, bird watching, bridge, backgammon, social dance, photography, gardening) **Treatment Directions** Assist the participant in the development and mastery of just one or two leisure skills which s/he can use upon discharge. Mastery of a few leisure skills does more then just allow the participant to engage in that activity. Mastery will help the participant develop increased confidence in himself/herself, an important step toward recovery. • Participation in recreational therapy groups that develop leisure skills • Participation in a variety of activities to develop foundation of skills (sports, games, play, hobbies)

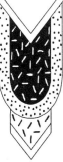

45

Problem	Goal	Treatment Directions
Lack of knowledge of home/community leisure resources	Increase knowledge in home and community resources	**Determining Functional Level** • Step 3 Part E of the **Leisure Step Up** • **Community Integration Program** (Armstrong and Lauzen 1994) Pre-test/Post-test Modules 1C (Basic Survival Skills), 2A (Theater), 2B (Restaurant), 2C (Library), 2D (Sporting Event), 3A (Shopping Mall), 3B (Grocery Store), 3C (Downtown), 3D (Bank), 3E (Laundromat), 4A (Personal Travel), 4B (Taxi/Taxi Vans), 4C (Train), 4D (Air Travel), 4E (City Bus) and 4F (Bus Station) • BUS Assessment (burlingame, 1989) **Treatment Directions** Ensure that the participant: 1. has the basic skills and knowledge to be able to locate the information that they need and/or 2. has the basic information written down and presented to him/her in such as way that s/he can use it. • Leisure resource groups using maps, brochures, newspapers, yellow pages of the phone book • Outings to the Chamber of Commerce, community visitor center • Community awareness field trips (bowling alleys, movie theaters, museums, zoos, libraries) • Leisure education groups (10 Things I love to do at home, 10 things I would take from my home if a tornado was coming) • Use of **LAFS: Leisure Activities Filing System** (Schenk, 1993)
Anhedonic (unable to receive pleasure from activities)	Receive/experience pleasure during/from leisure activities	**Determining Functional Level** • Leisure Attitude Scale (Beard and Ragheb, 1991) • Leisure Diagnostic Battery (Witt and Ellis, 1982) • Leisure Motivation Scale (Beard and Ragheb, 1989) • Leisure Satisfaction Scale (Beard and Ragheb, 1991) • Modified Beck Depression Inventory (Gallagher, 1979) • Free Time Boredom Measure (Ragheb and Meredith, 1994) **Treatment Directions** Identify the reason(s) that the participant is unable or unwilling to experience pleasure associated with leisure activities. It is likely that more than one issue will be inhibiting the participant's ability to enjoy his/her leisure activity. One issue to be sure to check for is depression (which may be a side effect of one or more medications). Once the therapist has been able to identify the reason(s) for the anhedonic affect, s/he should structure a treatment intervention. Do not overlook the importance of physical activity and exercise as a means to address anhedonic affect.

Problem	Goal	Treatment Directions
Lack of positive healthy leisure coping mechanisms	No participation in negative unhealthy leisure choices, participation in positive healthy leisure choices	**Determining Functional Level** • Coping Inventory for Stressful Situations (Endler and Parker, 1990) • Coping Operations Preference Enquiry (Schutz, 1962) • Coping Resources Inventory (Hammer and Marting, 1988) • Step 2 of Leisure Step Up **Treatment Directions** Determine how the participant copes with stress, how to make that coping more functional and then to assist the participant in the integration of healthy leisure activities to increase and maintain healthy coping mechanisms. • Educate the participant on the use of positive coping mechanisms (participation leisure coping mechanisms choices, participation in positive healthy choices in Step 2 — Leisure Plan, participation in activities) • Support the participant in making leisure choices followed by processing, counseling and leisure education • Basic needs being met by positive healthy leisure participation (belonging/love, gaining power and recognition, fun, being free, reality therapy needs) • Development of leisure attitudes, values, skills including classes, groups and community resources to teach skills, attitudes, values in various areas including arts, crafts, music, drama, dance, exercise, games, sports, physical activities, education, culture, collecting, volunteerism • Leisure assessments to define leisure ability • Refer to Treatment Directions Chart from other problem areas (leisure decision making, anhedonia, low self esteem, substance abuse) • Re-motivation leisure groups • Training in anger management, panic management, relaxation techniques and other specialized coping techniques which help address specific areas of need

47

Problem	Goal	Treatment Directions
Excessive use of leisure or workaholic	Identify reasons for unbalance in lifestyle Increase skill(s) in leisure (work) activities which the participant enjoys/finds pleasurable	**Determining Functional Level** • Contentment Scale (Bloom and Blenkner, 1970) • Days in My Life (Step 3D **Leisure Step Up**) • Leisure Attitude Scale (Beard and Ragheb, 1991) • Leisure Diagnostic Battery (Witt and Ellis, 1982) • Philadelphia Geriatric Center Morale Scale (Lawton, 1972) **Treatment Directions** Identify the pathology behind the unbalanced leisure or work lifestyle, then to address the specific deficits. It is unlikely that a "shotgun approach" to leisure education will work with these participants. Success in treatment will depend on the clear identification of the underlying causes. • Time management activities (Pie of Leisure Life, Days In My Life — Step 3D, counseling in leisure and living skills time management) • Recreational therapist and occupational therapist work together in written treatment plan • Education in values clarification (work ethic, monetary gains, family life, rest and relaxation) • Reference to Treatment Directions Chart from other problem areas (obsessive compulsive, low self esteem, lack of ability to express feelings, fear of failure/success, excessive guilt, family conflict) • Refer to psychotherapist, family counselor, co-dependent therapist, physician, other team members • Participate in relaxation therapy
Lack of leisure interests	Increase interests in leisure pursuits	**Determining Functional Level** • Leisure Interest Scale (Beard and Ragheb, 1991) • Leisurescope Plus (Schenk, 1993) • STILAP (Navar, 1990) • Free Time Boredom Measure (Ragheb and Meredith, 1994) **Treatment Directions** Determine what types of activities the participant enjoys (or has enjoyed in the past) and then set up a program for him/her to participate in activities of high interest and which are also practical and accessible for the participant. It is important to determine the cause of the lack of interest before treating the participant for a lack of interest in leisure. The lack of interest may be instead a lack of skills, a lack of experience with specific leisure activities or anhedonic tendencies. • Practical participation in high interest activities • Exploration past leisure interests and participation • Re-introduction activities of the past (**Leisure Step Up Step 5**)

48

Physical Domain

Problem	Goal	Treatment Direction
Lack of motivation/energy	Increase motivation and energy levels	**Determining Functional Level** • Leisure Motivation Scale (Beard and Ragheb, 1989) • Free Time Boredom Measure (Ragheb and Meredith, 1994) • Fitness assessment in areas of cardiovascular efficiency, muscular strength, muscular endurance flexibility (percent body fat as reported by dietitian) • Check medications — are the side effects possible cause of decreased motivation? **Treatment Directions** Because there are so many different causes for a lack of motivation and energy, the therapist needs to determine the cause of the lethargy before s/he can determine the direction that the treatment should take. Is the participant bored? Overwhelmed with responsibilities? Not feeling well or on medications that have decreased the participant's ability to be motivated? Once the therapist determines the source(s) of the problem, the process of addressing and correcting the problem can begin in earnest. • Therapeutic exercise/physical activity — cardiovascular exercise 2–6 times/week, within age-appropriate target heart rate zone (bicycling, walking, swimming, treadmill, stairmaster) *Be sure to have clearance from the participant's physician.* • Listening to "upbeat" music, motivating pictures and posters in appropriate areas (exercise room, kitchen, game room) • Promote appropriate sleeping patterns through activity and good dietary habits (active in afternoon, relaxing activities closer to bedtime, decaf drinks in evening) • No use of stimulus drugs besides prescriptions taken properly • Social contact with motivated, energetic peer group • Setting and accomplishing goals (short term, success oriented, healthy goals like walk a certain distance, complete craft project, write a letter) • Behavior modification techniques to reward desired, active behavior and ignore undesired, passive behavior as appropriate • Participate in leisure activities of personal interest • Education about leisure levels (Step 3 of **Leisure Step Up**)

Problem	Goal	Treatment Directions
Inappropriate somatic complaints	Decrease somatic complaints	**Determining Functional Level** • Results from testing done by other team members • Maladaptive Social Functioning Scale (1988) • Consult with physician on limitations **Treatment Directions** Work with the rest of the treatment team to determine the cause of the complaints, the severity of the condition and if the somatic complaints can be decreased with biofeedback and/or training in specific coping skills. • Modify therapeutic exercise or activity to not exacerbate somatic problems (stretching from a chair, walking, water aerobics) • Divert problem areas to positive healthy leisure participation • Muscle relaxation techniques (progressive muscle relaxation, massage) • Explore leisure interest with practical participation in areas of interest • Note leisure activity that precipitates the onset of pain, being careful not to reinforce inappropriate somatic behaviors • Leisure Plan from other problem areas (anxiety, lack of ability to express feelings, unmanageable stress, low self esteem)
Insomnia	Increase sleeping ability	**Determining Functional Level** • Interview with participant • Review of progress notes and nursing notes **Treatment Directions** Help the participant develop a routine which helps facilitate sleep. Do not overlook the possibility that the participant's inability to sleep is due to a side effect of one or more medications. • Consistent routine pattern of therapeutic exercise, physical activity, stretching, deep breathing (complete yogic breathing) • Relaxation techniques — both physical and mental • Appropriate diet and nutrition (no caffeine or other stimulants) • Relaxing leisure activities (hobbies, coloring, painting) • Relaxing reading material • Leisure Plan from other problem areas (stress, anxiety)

Problem	Goal	Treatment Directions
Substance Abuse	Total abstinence from drugs/alcohol Identify extent of problems that substance abuse is creating in the participant's life	**Determining Functional Level** • Step 3 of **Leisure Step Up** • Consult with Certified Addiction Counselor, Level 3 (CAC3) • Physical fitness assessment (cardiovascular efficiency, flexibility, muscular strength, muscular endurance, percent body fat) **Treatment Directions** Help the participant replace the old, unhealthy patterns of leisure with new, healthier ones that meet the needs that were met by substance abuse. • Alternative leisure pursuits (changing person, place and thing) or doing the old activities in a new way • Leisure counseling (Pie of Leisure Life, Step 3 of **Leisure Step Up** along with Step 5 to explore past issues) • Leisure skill development • Introduction of new leisure activities • Therapeutic exercise/physical activity to increase physical condition and decrease stress and craving • Reading educational material (AA Literature, spiritual daily meditation books, Adult Children of Alcoholics information) • Scheduling of structured and impromptu meetings – AA, NA, ACOA or other recovery support groups • Family leisure counseling • Making craft/art projects depicting themes (twelve step process, one day at a time, serenity prayer) • Attend church/religious organization • Participate in games/play (memory/cognitive games, addictionary, play it straight) • See Leisure Plan from other problem areas associated with substance abuse (self esteem, socialization/networking, communication skills, decision making) • Fitness prescription (YMCA, the Ys way to fitness or other established programs)

Problem	Goal	Treatment Directions
Eating disorders: obesity, anorexia, bulimia	Healthy eating, maintaining appropriate weight	**Determining Functional Level** • Interview with participant • Review of medical chart **Treatment Directions** Coordinate treatment with the rest of the treatment team using programming to increase appropriate body image, to sharpen reality orientation and to learn new patterns of leisure involvement. • Set goals for weight to achieve (reminder: one day/one meal at a time) • Be cautious about taking percent body fat if the diagnosis is bulimia or anorexia nervosa, as purging, binge eating or exercise patterns, may cause the percent body fat to seem high, adding to self image misconceptions • Leisure activity where person controls outcome (puzzles, crafts, building, making, shaping) • Leisure Plan from other problem areas (anger reduction, communication, trust, self image/self esteem, relaxation, social/family support) • Leisure skills, cooking groups, therapeutic exercise, physical activity (muscular strength for weight gain, aerobic for weight loss) *Consult physician on limitations.* • Leisure emotive, expressive groups, community outings (church/spiritual counseling, eating at a restaurant, support groups, Overeaters/Bulimic Anonymous) • Nutrition counseling, (food plan, what, how much, when) • Activities of high personal interest to decrease preoccupation with food and weight

Cognitive Domain

Problem	Goal	Treatment Directions
Lack of problem solving skills	Increase skills necessary to solve problems	**Determining Functional Level** • Observation of problem solving skills during activity • Wisconsin Card Sort or Trials Test (D. Grant and E. Berg, 1993) Usually given by psychologist **Treatment Directions** Increase the participant's skills in problem solving. Step 2 of the **Leisure Step Up** will help the participant increase his/her problem solving skills, since an important element of problem solving is to be able to identify where you are currently, where you want to be and select ways to get to where you want to go. • Understand basic steps in problem solving 1. identify the problem, 2. take responsibility to solve the problem, 3. list several possible solutions, 4. try the most likely solution, 5. if that solution doesn't work, try another solution • Play requiring low stress problem solving (knots exercise, new games, ropes course, killer) • Games requiring low stress problem solving (problem solver, computer games, puzzles, mazes, math games, untangle the nails, Rubic cubes, crosswords) • Home repairs requiring low stress problem solving (plumbing, woodworking, electrical, automobile) • Situational role play (role play solutions, empty chair)
Attention deficit	Increase attention span, focus, concentration	**Determining Functional Level** • There are many different aspects to attention deficit disorders. The psychiatrist can use some of his/her testing tools to pin point the specific aspects of the participant's disorder. **Treatment Directions** A participant may have many reasons for being unable to attend to the stimuli that s/he is supposed to. The therapist needs to identify the etiology of the deficit and direct treatment to compensate for the deficit. Treatment may be as simple as a behavior modification program using a rubber band around the participant's wrist. The participant snaps the rubber band if s/he notices his/her attention drifting. • Participation in high interest leisure activity • Participation in activity with attainable/foreseen goals (walk/run/jog given amount of distance, bowling, read a short story, archery, games like memory, war, concentration, Uno, speed) • Games with a timer (beat the clock, categories, taboo, Boggle Jr., Wordster) • Play needing attention for response (ping pong, tennis, badminton, speed bag) • Task oriented play — gradually increasing time frames — giving rest in between • Play gradually increasing amount of stimulus (larger room, increased population, more choices of play supplies)

53

Problem	Goal	Treatment Directions
Poor decision making skills	Increase decision making skills	**Determining Functional Level** • Interview with participant and review of participant's past decision making **Treatment Directions** Use a teaching system which helps the participant learn the step by step process of making decisions. The participant may also need to have some guidance and education as to what constitutes good decisions versus bad decisions. • Participant shares first in processing group therapy so s/he cannot copy others • Read a "choose your own adventure" book • Participant plans a leisure activity for self or group • Participate in Leisure Plan (Step 2 of **Leisure Step Up**) • Participate in creative, building, inventive, activities without directions (cooking with no recipe, block of clay, mixture of art/craft material) • Table games (chess, checkers, monopoly, strategy, assertion game, cribbage) • Play (human checkers, captain of team, football, horse basketball) • Unstructured leisure time (observe choices) • Participation in play in an assertive manner as opposed to passive or aggressive (involved as a participant, active, not allowing others to cheat, hurt, overpower them, not overly aggressive in taking advantage of game or participant)
Lack of recollection	Increase recent/remote memory	**Determining Functional Level** • Mini Mental State Test (Folstein, 1975) • Various reality orientation tests **Treatment Direction** Determine the cause of the participant's lack of recollection — is it a temporary condition, a progressive situation or a side effect of his/her medication? All interventions which aim at memory retention should work on having the participant learn the information by as many sensory inputs as possible. • Participation in stories, music, photos, personal items that are a part of the participant's past that would act as a catalyst to memory recall • Physical activity/exercise to stimulate thought process • Explore leisure of the past (Step 5 of **Leisure Step Up**, leisure education group) • Participation in games (memory, Simon Says, concentration, Trivial Pursuit) • Relaxation therapy (guided imagery recalling past) • Social conversation talking of childhood, looking for minute detail of events • Projects that require concentration, instruction, taking apart and rebuilding, following steps

Problem	Goal	Treatment Directions
Obsessive thoughts, compulsive behavior	Elimination of ritualistic behaviors	**Determining Functional Level** • Observation during activity • Results from testing done by other team members **Treatment Direction** Once the therapist and the participant have identified the type of problem rituals, use cognitive treatment to identify solutions and replace old behavior with new, frequently practiced, positive behaviors. • Provided structured schedule of activities to provide a feeling of security • Replace ritualistic behaviors with appropriate leisure participation. Initially begin with repetitive/play projects to relax uncontrollable rituals (latch-hook, beadwork, needle work, crochet, solitaire, Rubic cube, collection, target games) • Therapeutic exercise (stair climber, exercise bike, rowing machine) For participants who are frail, see **Safe Therapeutic Exercise for the Frail Elderly** by Hurley, 1988) • Relaxation therapy focused on relaxed, occupied thought — see **The Relaxation and Stress Reduction Workbook** by Davis, Robbins-Eshelman and McKay, 1988 • Emphasis on participation and pleasure in leisure activities, without emphasis on completion or competition (nature outings, picnics, swimming, entertainment) • Look also at problem areas of anxiety/stress or low self-esteem for leisure prescription ideas

Daily Living Skills

Problem	Goal	Treatment Directions
Unsafe living environment	To live in a safe environment	**Determining Functional Level** • Interview with participant • Reports by other team members **Treatment Directions** The directions for treatment depend on the etiology of the specific problems. • If the participant is unsafe due to abuse or threats in the home, consider a referral to the Department of Social Services, a social worker or a physician. • If the participant is unsafe due to a lack of cooking skills, telephone skills or personal hygiene, work on skills during leisure education time or refer to occupational therapist, physician, social worker. • If referrals are unavailable, work closely with nursing/treatment team to meet safety needs • Work with social worker to find safer neighborhood for participant • Teach safety and self defense skills
Poor personal health or hygiene	Improve self care	**Determining Functional Level** • Observation during activity • Results from testing by social work, occupational therapy, nursing **Treatment Direction** Assessment of personal care, followed by necessary skill development (bathing and showering, hair grooming, self care for wounds, clothes preparation, personal appearance, oral hygiene) • Change to exercise clothes for exercise and shower after exercise program or swimming • Work closely with nursing staff, occupational therapist, physical therapist, physician • Involvement in therapy group which works on good dressing and bathing skills • Teach participant to recognize when clean clothes and bathing are needed

Problem	Goal	Treatment Directions
Poor living skills	Functionality in living skills	**Determining Functional Level** • **Community Integration Program** Modules (Armstrong and Lauzen, 1994) Module 1A (Environmental Safety, Module 1B (Emergency Preparedness), Module 1C (Basic Survival Skills), Module 3A (Shopping Mall), Module 3B (Grocery Store), Module 3C (Downtown), Module 3D (Bank), Module 3E (Laundromat), Module 4A (Personal Travel), Module 5C (Leisure Activities) **Treatment Direction** Determine the specific deficits and their etiologies and then address the participant's needs with specific skills training. • Assessment in living skills, followed by skill development (cooking, cleaning, household tasks, money handling, food preparation, telephone tasks, transportation) • Daily schedule including all obligations, duties, leisure time • Group outings (arrange own transportation for leisure outing, order food at a restaurant, handle money, purchase items at store for cooking group, purchase toiletry items at a store) • Cooking/baking skill development (cooking group, nutrition education, food preparation, clean up) • Cleaning and disinfecting house, skills associated with household repairs, care of children/family (nutrition, clothing, hygiene, physical health and well being, discipline, grooming, teaching developmental skills) • Consult with occupational therapist, nutritionist, nursing staff

57

Problem	Goal	Treatment Directions
Lack of success with school or employment	Improve functionality in school/employment	**Determining Functional Level** • Assess Leisure Functioning that may be affecting school/job performance (substance abuse, negative peer influence, lack of sleep, poor nutrition) • Maladaptive Social Functioning Scale (1988) • Measurement of Social Empowerment and Trust (Witman, 1991) • School Social Behavior Scales (Merrell, 1993) • Cooperation and Trust Scale (Witman, 1991) • Comprehensive Evaluation in Recreational Therapy — Psych (Parker, 1989) **Treatment Directions** The therapist needs to identify the functional deficit(s) and the etiology of deficits before s/he can develop a specific intervention. • Exploration of fears/phobias associated with school/employment attendance/functionality • Participation in leisure outings to initiate re-entry in community/socialization as it can be less threatening and a lower expectation of performance • Consultation and information about skill level • Improve skill level (teacher/tutor involved, occupational therapist, social services/employment office, social worker) • Explore other problem areas (fear of failure/success, communication, socialization, self esteem, peer/authority conflicts) • Schedule leisure time to include time for homework, personal basic needs met through leisure

58

Social Domain

Problem	Goal	Treatment Directions
Peer/Authority conflicts	Minimize conflict with peer and authority figures	**Determining Functional Level** • Cooperation and Trust Scale (Witman, 1991) • Measurement of Social Empowerment and Trust Scale (Witman, 1991) • School Social Behavior Scale (Merrell, 1993) **Treatment Directions** Two of the primary sources for conflict are anger and mistrust. If the therapist can help the participant determine the reason for the conflict, strategies to ease the strain can be found. • Social skills group (1. conflict resolution skills training, 2. assertiveness skills training, 3. setting healthy limits and boundaries skills training) • Unstructured activity involving staff/authority, role play, cooperative play (new games, silver bullet) • Competitive play (sport activity, active games, table games with very clear rules to avoid conflict) • Anger management work • Adventure recreation (Outward Bound type programming)
Family conflict, parent/child conflict	Minimize conflict with family, enhance relationships	**Determining Functional Level** • Cooperation and Trust Scale (Witman, 1991) • Measurement of Social Empowerment and Trust Scale (Witman, 1991) **Treatment Directions** Two of the primary sources for conflict are anger and mistrust. If the therapist can help the participant determine the reason for the conflict, strategies to ease the strain can be found. In addition, the family group may need help in establishing boundaries, especially when the conflict involves a parent and adolescent. • Social skills group • Unstructured activity involving staff/authority, role play, cooperative play (new games, silver bullet) • Competitive play (sport activity, active games, table games where rules are followed to avoid conflict) • Anger management work • Adventure recreation (Outward Bound type programming) • Family leisure programming (participant's families attend functions, leisure education, family project, problem solving, play/games/activity) • Family role play • Family sculpturing • Therapeutic games (divorce cope, changing family game, talking, feeling and doing game, Ungame)

Problem	Goal	Treatment Directions
Lack of support systems	Develop network of support systems	**Determining Functional Level** • Family APGAR Scale (Smilkstein, 1978) **Treatment Directions** It is very hard for the therapist to help the participant establish a complete set of support systems within the participant's length of stay. The participant is most likely to connect with and follow through with support groups that s/he feels are of the greatest help. Determine the participant's perception for the type of support needed and build upon that. It takes significant social skills to stay engaged in a support system. The development of functional social skills may be indicated. • Socialization groups, (parties, events) • Small group settings (dyad/triad groups) • Recreational therapy socialization/play (team sports, cooperative play, dyad craft group) • Friendship groups (commonalties, likes, dislikes, sharing) • Therapeutic games (social security, Ungame, Halos-N-Horns, Assert with Love game) • Organizational activities (join clubs, church choir, youth group, cultural groups) • Volunteer activities (YMCA, YWCA, hospital, nursing homes, community agencies)
Lack of trust	Develop appropriate trust/trustworthy relationships	**Determining Functional Level** • Cooperation and Trust Scale (Witman, 1991) • Measurement of Social Empowerment and Trust (Witman, 1991) **Treatment Directions** Determine the aspect of trust that the participant has the greatest deficit in and then address that aspect (trust of one's own perception being correct, trust that others generally want to be trustworthy and trust that one can tell how trustworthy different participants are). • Trust exercises (blind nature walk, trust fall, trust lift) *Caution — only use these activities after trust is established to avoid harm to participant.* • Adventure groups that involve trust and cooperation (caving, ropes course, rappelling, rafting, climbing, hiking) • New games, play involving touch (tag, hug tag, freeze tag, twister, log walk, human spring/pyramid) • Basic trust may include building rapport through playing catch, dyad building project, ping pong, cards • Note that trust is an integral aspect of a therapeutic relationship between the therapist and the participant

Problem	Goal	Treatment Directions
Lack of communication skills	Increase ability to communicate	**Determining Functional Level** • Observation during activity • Results from testing done by other team members **Treatment Directions** Address skill development in one or two areas of communication at a time — allowing the participant to note improvement. Work with the rest of the team on a unified approach to social skill development. • Games and play (talking, feeling, doing game, Ungame, red rover, follow the leader, Simon Says, gossip game, pass the story game, communication blocks) • Games and play that incorporates eye contact between two or more participants • Discussion about talker/receiver/message • Team sports and play (football, water volleyball, soccer, team tag, hockey) • Team games (charades, Pictionary, password, communicate, bridge, Rook, trumps)
Social isolation	Decrease threatened state, increase socialization	**Determining Functional Level** • Comprehensive Evaluation in Recreational Therapy — Psych (Parker, 1989) • School Social Behavior Scale (Merrell, 1993) • Measurement of Social Empowerment and Trust (Witman, 1991) • Therapist's clinical judgment after observing participant in group activities **Treatment Directions** Increase the participant's awareness of his/her need for socialization — how it will help him/her feel better. The actual skills required to develop and maintain friendships are extremely complex skills requiring training in specific techniques. • Opportunities for socialization with brief, frequent visits by the recreational therapist for play/activity (dominos, cards, checkers, craft activity, building models, knitting, drawing, painting) • Increasing communication and play socialization (eye contact, verbalization, body language, interaction, touch) • Increasing amounts of time, gradually involving others in relaxed/unstructured leisure (watching TV/movie, free play in game room, entertainment) • Slowly introducing increased cooperation and socialization (sing-a-long, ice cream social, cooking/baking) • Increasing structure (team participation, Pictionary, password, ping pong, volleyball, story telling, dancing) • Increase involvement with participant initiating interaction • Refer to other problem areas and their prescriptions (trust, anxiety, fears, communication, obsessive thoughts)

61

Psychological Domain

Problem	Goal	Treatment Directions
Pre-occupation with problem areas	Decrease pre-occupation with problem	**Determining Functional Level** • Mini Mental State Examination (Folstein, 1975) • Observe participant's behaviors during activity **Treatment Directions** For a participant who has difficulty with pre-occupation in his/her problem areas the therapist needs to help him/her develop self-directed thought control through the use of standardized programs and techniques. • Relaxation therapy (guided imagery, subliminal messages) • Therapeutic exercise and physical activity • Reading/movie (emotionally involved story, high interest material, plot needing much concentration) • Practical project requiring much attention (pin stripe painting, detail work, step by step instruction, leather craft) • Games (concentration, memory, clue, chess, Simon Says, word games, Scrabble) • Leisure activity of high enjoyment
Fear of failure or success	Decrease fear, increase acceptance of failure and success	**Determining Functional Level** • Through interview and observation try to determine family messages given about failure and success • Observe participant's threshold for frustration and how s/he deals with failure and success **Treatment Directions** Address the functional skills lost as a result of the participant's reactions to frustration, poor self image and perceptions of weakness. Generally, supporting the participant through the development of skills in a single leisure activity to the point that s/he can achieve success and, with the support of the therapist, react to success appropriately is a good direction to take. • Goal setting (reach Target Heart Rate Zone in therapeutic exercise, complete a hobby project, climb a mountain) • Identification of positive leisure abilities • Participate as a spectator in competitive event and process experience • Participate in competition and process experience (human checkers, Pictionary, world wide games) • Explore past leisure experiences (**Leisure Step Up, Step 5**) • Counseling in value of leisure expression, not competition (winning or losing)

Problem	Goal	Treatment Directions
Unmanageable stress, anxiety, panic attacks	No panic attacks, minimize anxiety, stress in control	**Determining Functional Level** • Observation of participant during activity • Results from the tests given by the other team members **Treatment Directions** Work on desensitization training and/or stress reduction training. The participant may need to change the approach that s/he takes to activities to reduce symptoms. • Relaxing leisure activity (painting, playing a musical instrument, nature outing, bird watching, star gazing, journalizing, coloring, watching fish in a fish tank, horticulture, singing) • Relaxation therapy (progressive muscle relaxation, deep breathing, guided imagery, meditation, prayer) • Therapeutic exercise and physical activity (stretching, aerobic activity, swimming, walking, full range of motion) • Intense laughter and music therapy • Take participant out of affective mode, into cognitive mode (Rubic cube, card games, trivial pursuit, Nintendo) • Positive escape activities (movies, story telling, reading a magazine) • Therapeutic table games (Stress Attack, Stress Strategies, Coping)
Lack of ability to express feelings	To freely express feelings through leisure	**Determining Functional Level** • Observation of participant during activities **Treatment Directions** Work on the basic skills associated with communication with self and/or others in an environment where the participant feels both emotionally and physically safe. • Use art, nature, music, drama, dance, pet therapies, journalizing, poetry, writing • Games/play (feelings, charades, feelings in hand, dealing with feelings) • Participation in leisure activities of positive healthy choices (Step 3A — **Leisure Levels of Leisure Step Up**), therapeutic exercise, physical activity, creative, inventive and imaginative activities • Psychodrama

Problem	Goal	Treatment Directions
Inappropriate flat affect	Heighten expression, decrease depression	**Determining Functional Level** • Observation of participant during activities — both group and one on one • Results from testing done by the other team members **Treatment Directions** Teach the participant to identify his/her inappropriate affect and to provide the participant with opportunities to practice using appropriate affects. • Participate in pleasurable activity • Movement therapy • Therapeutic exercise (stretching, aerobic, muscular strength) • Laughter (joke book, movie, pictures, funny songs) • Pet therapy • Full range of motion • Gross motor activity (darts, walking, gardening, parachute games, golf, baseball, badminton, racquetball) • Nature and outings (camping, hiking, backpacking, bird watching, fishing, picnics, horseback riding, gardening, barbecuing) • Activities using senses (cooking, baking, skiing, music, outside activities, crafts, hobbies) • Psychodrama • Play therapy • Religious/spiritual activities (group prayer meetings, Bible study, outreach)

Problem	Goal	Treatment Directions
Delusions, hallucinations	Improve reality functioning	**Determining Functional Level** • Observation during activity • Results from the testing by other members of the treatment team **Treatment Directions** For hallucinations, redirect the participant to pay attention to the here-and-now of the activity using reality orientation techniques throughout the session. For delusional activity, engage the participant in highly structured, tactile and sensory motor based activities limited to 30 minutes in duration. • Participation in simple, concrete, low stimulus activity (small-group catch with a Frisbee or ball unless flying objects present a problem) • Table games (checkers, world wide games, ping pong, card games, dominos) • Stay away from therapeutic games (coping and decisions, addictionary, Ungame, assert with love) • Stay away from abstract thought, meditation/guided imagery, delusional issues, feelings, verbal expression, self awareness • Provide a safe environment • Reinforce taking prescribed medications • Participate in reality oriented program (personal hygiene, making bed, brushing teeth) • Re-focus participant back to reality of present time, place and date
Low self esteem	Exhibit positive self esteem	**Determining Functional Level** • Social Empowerment and Trust Scale (Witman, 1991) • Observation during activity **Treatment Directions** Help the participant to be able to acknowledge his/her strengths as s/he gains strength in a specific activity. • Successful completion of project (puzzle, hobby, **Leisure Step Up Workbook**, reading a book, home repair, car repair, collecting activities) • Success in play (strike in bowling, hit the target, pop the balloon, kick the ball, ski down the hill) • New activity skill development • Achieve goal (walk 2 miles, complete homework, climb the mountain) • Mirror therapy (look at self while exercising, putting on make-up) • Positive thoughts of affirmations during leisure activity or relaxing (I can hit the ball, I will learn this skill, I am participating fine) • Therapeutic table games (self concept, self-esteem)

Problem	Goal	Treatment Directions
Oppositional defiant behaviors/conduct disorders	Self directed appropriate behavior	**Determining Functional Level** • School Social Behavior Scale (Merrell, 1993) • Comprehensive Evaluation in Recreational Therapy — Psych (Parker, 1989) **Treatment Directions** Assist the participant in learning appropriate boundaries and consequences for his/her behaviors. Coping skills, problem solving and relaxation techniques may be an important part of the participant's treatment program. • Games/play with boundaries and consequences enforced • Play (freeze tag, basketball, soccer, tennis, hockey, volleyball, walleyball) • Games (horseshoes, ping pong, Sorry, Trouble, dominos, computer games, problem solving game) • Activity that cannot be manipulated (overnight camping/survival outings, as one cannot manipulate the weather, no cooking/no eating, follow the rules or natural consequences occur) • Weight training — either the weights get lifted or they do not, they cannot be manipulated, rowing machine, exercise bike with computer readout • Community outings (staff to observe behaviors and to be role models) • Behavioral modification being enforced during leisure • Leisure activities that involve true leadership (caving, cross-country skiing, rappelling, rock climbing) • Religious/spiritual involvement (church choir, meditation group, outreach services)
Out of control anger or rage	No rage outbursts, anger used appropriately as a motivator	**Determining Functional Level** • Observation during activity • Results from other team member's evaluations **Treatment Directions** Help the participant develop skills in anger management, stress reduction and, importantly, not to use their body when they are angry. (These participant's frequently use their bodies as weapons when they are angry.) • Therapeutic exercise (speed bag, vigorous aerobic activity within target heart rate zone, weight training) • Relaxation technique (progressive muscle relaxation, guided imagery, visualization) • Soft music (sometimes loud music is relaxing to teens) • Active play/games (racquetball, soccer, x-country skiing, tennis, bicycling, basketball) • Emotive expression (drawing, coloring, painting, lacing, tearing paper, poetry, pottery, leather crafts, singing) *Use these activities when the participant is not actively engaged in anger or rage.* • Psychodrama

References

Armstrong, M. and S. Lauzen. 1984. **Community Integration Program**. Ravensdale. Idyll Arbor, Inc. (206) 432-3231. e-mail IdyArbor@ix.netcom.com

Beard, J. and M. Ragheb. 1991. *Idyll Arbor Leisure Battery*. Ravensdale. Idyll Arbor, Inc. (206) 432-3231. e-mail IdyArbor@ix.netcom.com

Beard, J. and M. Ragheb. 1991. *Leisure Attitude Measurement*. Ravensdale. Idyll Arbor, Inc. (206) 432-3231. e-mail IdyArbor@ix.netcom.com

Beard, J. and M. Ragheb. 1991. *Leisure Interest Measurement*. Ravensdale. Idyll Arbor, Inc. (206) 432-3231. e-mail IdyArbor@ix.netcom.com

Beard, J. and M. Ragheb. 1989. *Leisure Motivation Scale*. Ravensdale. Idyll Arbor, Inc. (206) 432-3231. e-mail IdyArbor@ix.netcom.com

Beard, J. and M. Ragheb. 1991. *Leisure Satisfaction Measure*. Ravensdale. Idyll Arbor, Inc. (206) 432-3231. e-mail IdyArbor@ix.netcom.com

Beck, A., C.H. Ward, M. Mendelson, J. Mock and J. Erbaugh. 1961. "An Inventory for Measuring Depression" *Archives of General Psychiatry* 4 (1961):53-63, as modified by D. Gallagher, Andrus Gerontology Center, University of Southern California, 1979.

Bloom, M. and M. Blenkner. 1970. "Assessing Functioning of Older Persons Living in the Community" *The Gerontologist* 10 (1970):331-337.

burlingame, j. 1989. *Bus Utilization Skills Assessment (BUS)*. Idyll Arbor, Inc. (206) 432-3231. e-mail IdyArbor@ix.netcom.com

Davis, Robins-Eshelman and McKay. 1988. **The Relaxation and Stress Reduction Workbook — Third Edition**. Oakland. New Harbinger Publications. *Available through* Idyll Arbor, Inc. (206) 432-3231. e-mail IdyArbor@ix.netcom.com

Endler, N. and J. Parker. 1990. *Coping Inventory for Stressful Situations (CISS)*. Ontario. Multi-Health Systems, Inc. (416) 424-1700.

Folstein, M. S. Folstein and P. McHugh. 1975. "Mini-Mental State: A Practical Method for Grading the Cognitive State of Patients for the Clinician" *Journal of Psychiatric Research* 12 (1975):55-67.

Grant, D. and E. Berg (1993). *Wisconsin Card Sorting Test (WCST)*. Odessa. Psychological Assessment Resources. (813) 968-3003.

Hammer, A. and M. Marting. 1988. *Coping Resources Inventory (CRI)*. Palo Alto. Consulting Psychologists Press, Inc. (415) 969-8901

Hurley, O. 1988. **Safe Therapeutic Exercise for the Frail Elderly: An Introduction**. Albany. The Center for the Study of Aging. *Available through* Idyll Arbor, Inc. (206) 432-3231. e-mail IdyArbor@ix.netcom.com

Lawton, M. 1972. "Dimensions of Morale" **Research Planning and Action for the Elderly**, ed. D. Kent, R. Kastenbaum and S. Sherwood. New York. Behavioral Publications.

Maladaptive Social Functioning Scale. 1988. *Available through* Idyll Arbor, Inc. (206) 432-3231. e-mail IdyArbor@ix.netcom.com

Merrell, K. 1993. *School Social Behavior Scales.* Brandon. Clinical Psychology Publishing. *Available through* Idyll Arbor, Inc. (206) 432-3231. e-mail IdyArbor@ix.netcom.com

Navar, N. 1990. *STILAP (1990).* Idyll Arbor, Inc. (206) 432-3231. e-mail IdyArbor@ix.netcom.com

Parker, R. 1975 — Revised 1989 and 1994. *Comprehensive Evaluation in Recreational Therapy —Psych.* Ravensdale. Idyll Arbor, Inc. (206) 432-3231. e-mail IdyArbor@ix.netcom.com

Ragheb, M. and S. Meredith. 1995. *Free Time Boredom Measure.* Ravensdale. Idyll Arbor, Inc. (206) 432-3231. e-mail IdyArbor@ix.netcom.com

Schenk, C. 1993. **LAFS Plus: Leisure Activities Filing System**. Tallahassee. Leisure Dynamics. *Available through* Idyll Arbor, Inc. (206) 432-3231. e-mail IdyArbor@ix.netcom.com

Schenk, C. 1993. *Leisurescope Plus.* Tallahassee. Leisure Dynamics. *Available through* Idyll Arbor, Inc. (206) 432-3231. e-mail IdyArbor@ix.netcom.com

Schenk, C. 1993. *Teen Leisurescope Plus.* Tallahassee. Leisure Dynamics. *Available through* Idyll Arbor, Inc. (206) 432-3231. e-mail IdyArbor@ix.netcom.com

Schutz, W. 1962 *Coping Operations Preference Enquiry (COPE).* Palo Alto. Mind Garden, Inc. (415) 424-8493 e-mail MindGarden@eworld.com

Smilkstein, G. 1978. "The Family APGAR: A Proposal for a Family Function Test and Its Use by Physicians" *Journal of Family Practice* 6 (1978): 1231-1239.

Sweetland, R. and D. Keyser. 1991. **Tests: A Comprehensive Reference for Assessments in Psychology, Education and Business**. Austin. PRO-ED, Inc. (512) 451-3246.

Wessel, J. 1979. **ICAN: Sport, Leisure and Recreation Skills**. Austin. PRO-ED, Inc. (512) 451-3246

Witman, J. 1991. *Cooperation and Trust Scale.* Ravensdale. Idyll Arbor, Inc. (206) 432-3231. e-mail IdyArbor@ix.netcom.com

Witman, J. 1991. *Measurement of Social Empowerment and Trust.* Ravensdale. Idyll Arbor, Inc. (206) 432-3231. e-mail IdyArbor@ix.netcom.com

Witt, P. and G. Ellis. 1982. *Leisure Diagnostic Battery.* State College. Venture Publishing. (814) 234 4561. e-mail VPublish@pipeline.com

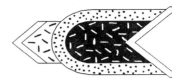 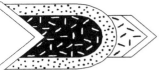

Step 3
Leisure Education

Step 3 — Leisure Education gives the participant important information about leisure which is necessary for a healthy lifestyle. Step 3 consists of 6 parts: Participation in part or in all of the aspects of Leisure Education will give the participant and the therapist added information and a better understanding about the participant's leisure.

    A)   An understanding of the Leisure Level Model. Part A will educate the participant in positive and negative leisure behaviors.

    B)   Leisure Participation Level. Part B will give information regarding the participant's leisure participation level.

    C)   Leisure Attitude Awareness Stems. Part C will identify the participant's attitude toward leisure participation.

    D)   Days In My Life. Part D will identify the participant's use of time during a typical 24 hour day.

    E)   Leisure Resources. Part E will educate the participant in basic home and community leisure resources.

    F)   Things I Enjoy. Part F will identify the participant's leisure interests and areas of enjoyment.

The form on the following page can be used to document the completion of each part of Step 3. Following the form are further descriptions of each of the parts of Step 3.

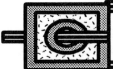

Step 3 Checklist

Name _____   **Date** _____

Directions: Use this checklist to keep track of the parts of Step 3.

A) The Leisure Level Model. Part A will tell you about positive and negative leisure behaviors.

      Completed _____

B) Leisure Participation Level. Part B will give you information about your leisure participation level.

      Completed _____

C) Leisure Attitude Awareness Stems. Part C will help you understand your attitude toward leisure activities.

      Completed _____

D) Days In My Life. Part D will identify your use of time during a typical 24 hour day.

      Completed _____

E) Leisure Resources. Part E will tell you about basic home and community leisure resources.

      Completed _____

F) Things I Enjoy. Part F will identify your leisure interests and areas of enjoyment.

      Completed _____

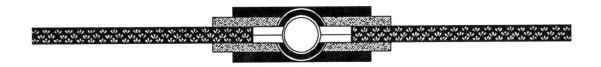

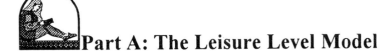 Part A: The Leisure Level Model

This step requires the participant to gain an understanding and knowledge of the Leisure Level Model. The recreational therapist can help the participant gain an understanding by presenting the material in a 1:1 or group therapy fashion. The format is simple if the presenter has a clear understanding of the concept. When they see the model, many participants realize for the first time that what they do makes a difference. They say things like "It really does make a difference what I do with my free time" and "I didn't realize that being creative helped me express my feelings", "I guess being in a gang really is negative."

In presenting the following material:
   1) Explain the format of the Leisure Level Model.
   2) Define or ask the participants to define leisure, free time, recreation.
   3) Explain that each level begins with My Choices/My Behaviors.
   4) Use visual aids.
   5) Begin explaining at Level 0 and work your way down, then go to Level 1 and work your way up.
   6) Explain each level thoroughly giving examples of each.
   7) Point out the differences of each level (even though two people can participate at the same activity, the manner determines the level).
   8) Explain unhealthy, negative choices (rebound effect/consequences) and healthy positive changes (emotive expressive/benefits).

The Leisure Level Model

The Leisure Level Model explains various levels of activity participation. It consists of nine different levels, three of which are negative, one neutral and five positive. The higher the level the more potential positive health benefit the participant receives. Participation in Levels 2, 3, 4 and Cathartic Level are emotive expressive levels, in that feelings are expressed with participation. This is particularly important in therapy, as many people have difficulty with verbal expression and need a way to express themselves. Participation in the upper levels is considered a healthy leisure lifestyle with healthy benefits. Activities in Levels 2, 3, 4 and Cathartic Level are those that we, as therapists, should prescribe in Step 2, the Leisure Plan. Participation in Levels -1, -2 and lost freedom are negative choices. The lower the level the more severe the negative unhealthy consequence. The unhealthy consequence is known as the negative rebound effect. In that, it has repercussions that will follow, leading eventually to being unhealthy. This outcome affects the individual negatively and may also affect the individual's family, social network and community.

There are many definitions for the terms free time, recreation and leisure. The three terms are generally considered the same and are used synonymously by the non-professional, but there are differences which will help the participant understand his/her situation better.

Free Time: A block or amount of time that we are free to do what we choose.

Recreation: What we choose to do during free time. This term is often mistaken for relaxing time.

Leisure: A frame of mind where we are able to enjoy the activities that we are doing; to find pleasure and to have our needs met.

Most individuals do not include unhealthy negative choices as part of Leisure Participation, it is important to point this out as it brings individual responsibility to the participant's choices and behaviors.

The following pages give descriptions of each of the levels of leisure participation. All of the levels begin with the words *My Choices/My Behavior.* This is to reinforce the ideas of freedom of choice in leisure and that choices lead to the individual's behavior. This is extremely important in therapy, as our choices are a determining factor in becoming healthy or unhealthy. There are three aspects in how we spend our life: working (including basic activities of daily living), leisure (and advanced activities of living) and sleep. All aspects of life offer choice to the individual. Leisure however, offers a greater opportunity (and many times availability) in getting our needs met. With true leisure participation there is no obligation, duty or outside reward. Leisure activities are voluntary and intrinsic.

Reality therapy states that we have four basic psychological needs:

1) Belonging (living, cooperating)
2) Power (competing, achieving, gaining importance)
3) Freedom (moving, choosing)
4) Fun (learning, playing)

and if our needs are met with flexible effective behaviors, we will have a successful identity, have effective control of our life, be strong, responsible and self disciplined. Leisure participation offers the opportunity to get many of our basic needs met.

In explaining the Leisure Level Model, a visual aid is extremely helpful, as it enables the participant to see the levels stepping upward or falling off a cliff. Having a large model on the wall and one in front of the individual makes explanation and understanding an easier process. An overhead projector or drawing on a chalkboard will suffice for the large model. The following pages are included in the handout for each participant.

You must be sensitive to the feelings of the participant that is given this information. The lost freedom category may provoke strong feelings if the participant is in a situation where s/he has experienced a loss of freedom. If the participant is not capable of reading and understanding the material, you will need to present the information in a way that s/he can understand it.

Leisure Level Model

The activities that I choose to participate in during my free time.

Healthy Positive Choices ⇒ ⇒ ⇒ ⇒

Unhealthy Negative Choices ⇐ ⇐ ⇐ ⇐

Cathartic Level

My Choices/My Behavior. My participation reaches a point of catharsis. My participation makes a measurable change in my life. **Examples:** vacation, climbing a mountain, prayer, ropes course, watching an event, achieving the goal, etc.

Level 4

My Choices/My Behavior. I am creative, inventive, imaginative, taking nothing and making something. Not following a plan or instruction. **Examples:** Poetry, drawing, painting, crafts, cooking, sculpting, music, prayer, etc.

Level 3

My Choices/My Behavior. I am active physically, socially and/or cognitively. Activity follows instruction, a plan, rules, with participation on an emotional level. **Examples:** Crafts, cooking, bike riding, sports participation, intense laughter (internal jogging), dancing, games, skateboarding, reading, physical workout, relaxation therapy, etc.

Level 2

My Choices/My Behavior. I am a spectator emotionally involved. There is a personal investment, true entertainment. **Examples:** TV, radio, watching others participate in Level 3 and 4 activities.

Level 1

My Choices/My Behavior. I am a spectator with no emotional involvement. Participation lacks personal investment, *positive* activities with nothing else to do. **Examples:** Watching TV, listening to the radio, watching others participate in Level 3 and 4 activities.

Level 0

My Choices/My Behavior. Participation could be forced, obligated, duty, with no internalization of participation. Preoccupation during participation in Level 3 or 4 activities.

Level -1

My Choices/My Behavior. I am preoccupied in thought or feeling and just going through the motions of the activity. Participation in Level 1, 2, 3 or 4 activities.

Level -2

My Choices/My Behavior. I am harmed physically, mentally or emotionally. **Examples:** Substance abuse, dangerous high risk activities, self abuse, negative thinking, poor dietary choices, too much or not enough sleeping, eating, exercising, relaxing, etc.

Lost Freedom

My Choices/My Behavior. I affect others in a harmful or hurting manner. This includes physical, emotional or mental harm to my family, friends or community. **Examples:** Substance abuse, inappropriate competition, gossip, threatening, name calling, fighting, hurting animals, breaking the law (minor), no family time, etc.

My Choices/My Behavior. I harm myself or others. My behavior causes a loss in freedom to choose my own leisure. Often the victim's and/or family's leisure are also affected. **Examples:** Crime, gang involvement, vandalism, fighting, suicide gestures, breaking the law (major: rape, self abuse, sexual abuse, substance abuse, etc.).

Explanation of the Leisure Levels

Level 0: Preoccupied

Level 0 is neither a positive or a negative level. It is when you are pre-occupied in thought or feeling and will get little to no benefits from participating in an upper level activity.

When your thoughts or feelings are not connected with what you are doing, you are not really "into" the activity. You are there physically, but nothing else. Pre-occupation many times is on work, problem areas, responsibilities, things you think you really should be doing, feelings of guilt, depression, anger, frustration, etc.

An example that you might identify with: Suppose you go on a weekend vacation (to a fantastic place) but the whole time you are there you are pre-occupied about a poor relationship, fear of what could happen during the weekend, worrying about past abuse issues, etc. You might as well have stayed home, since you are functioning on Level 0 and are not really mentally and emotionally at this fantastic place.

You may also be participating at Level 0 when you are forced to do something by outside pressure or influence. An example of this: you feel obligated to attend a family function that you do not wish to attend. It may be a duty or you may feel forced. Because of this pressure you may not internalize the participation, thus you are participating at Level 0.

An exception to this would be if you are pre-occupied with a problem area, solving or partially solving the problem during leisure participation. Problem solving during leisure is participation on a therapeutic level. For example, if you take the weekend vacation to a fantastic place and it solves or deals with a problem about a poor relationship, fear of the unknown, past abuse issues, etc., then you are participating on a therapeutic level which is extremely positive and healthy. Other examples include: 1) engaging in physical activity or exercise when you are pre-occupied with anger, hurt, frustration, etc. and you release feelings through participation; 2) engaging in poetry, story writing, journalizing, art, crafts, music, etc. to express or deal with problem areas; 3) watching a movie, reading a book, listening to a song, etc., vicariously solving your problems through emotional involvement as a spectator.

The therapeutic level is the outcome of the Leisure Plan from Step 2. It is the difference between leisure participation in drama and therapeutic participation in psychodrama. The difference between social talking in a group and a group therapy session. The difference between talking with someone and a therapeutic individual session. The difference between a family talking and a therapeutic family session. It is truly getting your needs met by solving problems.

Level -1: Harm To Myself

Level -1 is the first level in the unhealthy negative direction. It is when your participation during leisure is harmful to yourself. There may not be an initial problem created by participation, but if you continue, you will eventually be less healthy. Examples of this include smoking cigarettes, eating junk food, lack of activity, etc. Another example, would be when you participate in an activity such as bowling, skiing, crafts, etc. with negative thoughts such as: I'm dumb, I'll never learn how to do this, I always look stupid trying something new, I must be the dumbest person here, etc.

A key factor in this level is too much or not enough. Often times it is difficult to determine how much is too much or how little is too little. A good rule of thumb is, if doing something causes you trouble — even a little bit, it is probably a Level -1 activity. Some examples might be watching a violent movie, reading an over stimulating sex book, listening to negative messages in music, etc. Often participation in these activities lead to Level -2 or Lost Freedom.

Keep in mind that you need to be very careful not to say something is okay for you when it really isn't. Your therapist and others around you may be seeing it more clearly than you are.

Level -2: Harm To Others
Level -2 is the second level of unhealthy negative choices. At times your participation on Level -1 will fall to Level -2 as the ways you are hurting yourself start to hurt others. Examples include: addictions to drugs, alcohol, gambling, sex or work which harms members of your family. A good test for whether you are harming others is not what you think, but how others tell you they feel. It's hard to admit to yourself that you are hurting the ones you love, but if they say it is so, you should at least admit that it might be true.

You might consider participation on this level as fun, exciting or a means of self expression. This can be true, but if your actions also hurt others, they are unhealthy and negative. Sooner or later they will bring harm and hurt to you or others. Having fun at someone else's expense is also a poor choice in leisure. Examples include: ethnic jokes, stealing, destruction of property, gossip and lying about an individual. These are all Level -2 activities.

Lost Freedom
Lost Freedom cannot be given a negative number, as even participation in positive levels cannot balance your leisure life. Participation on this level has a drastic effect upon you and others affected by your behavior. It is extremely important for you to have a clear understanding of this level if you have experienced this level first hand, either as a participant or as a victim.

If you participate on this level, you may lose your freedom by having to deal with consequences such as negative self feelings, thoughts and self esteem. You are not locked into this level and through therapeutic intervention you may change your leisure lifestyle and deal with issues causing your behaviors. Examples include: harm from drunk driving, rape, serious injury due to fighting, going to prison for stealing, etc.

If you have been a victim of a violent action, you may also be on this level, especially if you experience extreme feelings of fear, guilt, anger, along with thoughts of low self esteem, lack of interest or vindictiveness. Being a victim of violence has a tremendous effect on your freedom in choosing leisure. Therapeutic intervention may restore your positive thoughts and feelings, enabling you to choose of a healthy leisure lifestyle.

You are also participating at this level if you are pre-occupied with suicidal thoughts, involved in self abuse or suicidal gestures. Violent acts against yourself cloud your mind and decision making ability, limiting your freedom to make healthy/positive leisure choices. Examples: cutting oneself with a razor blade, suicide attempts, pre-occupation with extreme negative and suicidal thought, gang fighting with no self concern, sexual promiscuity with no protection, etc. Therapeutic intervention is helpful and many times necessary to help you regain a healthy leisure lifestyle.

Level 1: Uninvolved Spectator

Level 1 participation is on the low end of positive healthy participation. When you first look at this level, it may appear of little value. There are, however, times when your mind, body and emotions are fatigued and you need to do nothing. Our culture has stringent demands for both work and play and it can be hard for you to do nothing (and not feel guilty). You are on this level if you are a spectator with no emotional investment. Examples are watching cars drive by while sitting on the porch, resting while listening to background music, attending a sporting event with no concern for outcome, etc.

Level 2: Involved Spectator

Level 2 is similar to Level 1, except that you are emotionally involved as a spectator. You are on this level when you are interested and experiencing or expressing an emotion. Examples are going to a sad movie, reading a dramatic book, watching a love story on TV, attending an emotionally charged basketball game, attending a museum with a high interest in the art work, etc. You must be careful in this area, as we live in a society that wants to be entertained. TV, for example, monopolizes many lives. If you spend all of your time watching TV (or playing Nintendo), you are on Level -1 not Level 2. Too much TV or Nintendo is just not good for you.

Level 3: Active Participation

Level 3 participation is an upper level in the Leisure Level Model continuum. When defining recreation most people think of activity on this level. If you are on this level you are a player, a participant as opposed to a spectator as in Levels 1 and 2. It includes cognitive, physical and social parts. You need to think. You need to move your body. You need to interact with others. And you need to be able to perform tasks requiring significant levels of coordination. One is not a substitute for the other, as we must participate in some element of physical, social and cognitive activity on a regular basic to be healthy. A key point in this level is following a plan, instruction or rules during participation.

The physical category is extremely important in therapy and needs to be a part of all of our lives in maintaining health. Physical activity and exercise may be the most used and highly accepted therapeutic programming approach in recreational therapy. If you have been inactive or if you are in poor physical condition, you must be careful when you start to do more physical exercise. Talk with your doctor before you begin an exercise program. Examples of physical participation include: riding a bike, fly fishing, weight training, walking a nature trail, following an instructor in aerobic exercise, playing racquetball, jogging or dancing the fox-trot.

The cognitive category includes the thinking process. Your participation in cognitive aspects are important because thinking clearly is important in solving problems. Participation in cognitive activities sharpens our thought process leading to improved decision making, listening skills, improved memory, etc. Examples of cognitive participation are reading a "how to" repair book, playing a game of strategy, chess, Clue, Memory, reminiscing while watching home movies, working on puzzles, math problems, word problems or following instructions in building a model ship.

The social category includes verbal and/or non-verbal conversation/interaction with at least one other person. Your participation must include emotional involvement or the socialization would be on a lower level. You may think sitting down with a friend and carrying on a conversation or being at a party or engagement with a group as the only way to be social. Socialization also includes non-verbal participation in recreation activities. The action, the play, the movement are your means of communication. Examples include playing checkers, basketball, table games, sport activity and group projects.

It is not necessarily important to decide if an activity is physical, social or cognitive. The decision however would be which aspects are considered important during participation.

For a healthy leisure you need to have some of each. How you mix and match your activities to get them all is ultimately up to you.

Level 4: Creative Participation

Level 4 participation offers a means of expressing your emotions. It is above Level 3 in emotive expression, in that your participation does not follow a plan, pattern or instruction. You leave part of yourself in what you accomplish and what you accomplish becomes part of you. Many poets, artists and musicians describe this level of participation as including their soul, the essence of their existence. A key phrase is taking nothing and making something. Examples are taking a lump of clay and molding a figure, writing a short story, cooking from scratch (no recipe), talking to God from your heart, making plans to decorate for a party or unstructured free play.

Contrary to what you may believe, this level can be achieved by learning and practicing. Some people say, "I'm not a creative person." However, creativity can be learned. Just like all good things, it takes work (or play, depending on your perception of leisure) to be successfully creative.

Cathartic Level: Growth Through Participation

Cathartic Level is the ultimate level in leisure participation. It is free time participation that is extremely emotional. When you are participating in Level 2, 3 or 4 activities, you may reach a cathartic point. It is your personal growth that many times acts as a catalyst for a change in your lifestyle. Many times you cannot plan to achieve this level. It happens as a result of the right chemistry of your emotional state and the activity. It is participation on a Level 2, 3 or 4 that has a lasting and memorable effect on you. Examples are watching a movie that portrays an aspect your life teaching you new values, talking to God and gaining inspiration, going on a family vacation that solidifies family ties.

Summary

The Leisure Level Model is a tool that gives value to choices and behaviors during leisure time. It can help you see that what you do with your leisure time does make a difference and it gives you a goal to achieve. You do not always need to participate on a high level. You need to find a balance among the positive Levels 1 through 4, while staying away from participation on the negative levels.

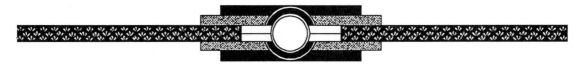

 Part B: Leisure Participation Level

The Leisure Participation Level gives the participant the basic idea of the quality in which s/he chooses to live his/her free time. Column A is for activities that the person has participated in within the last 30 days. It may be difficult to recall the exact participation for the last 30 days but most participants will recall the essentials. (Thirty days is used because that time frame will serve as an indicator to the participant's current mental health status. Those needing counseling will generally have precipitating events within their lifestyle that are indicative of their needing treatment.) The Leisure Level Model (Column B) shows the points the participant receives. Note that both positive and negative participation are included. Column C is used to record the number of times the listed activity has been participated in within the given time frame. Column D is the subtotal of all positive and negative activities (multiplying Column B times Column C). A Grand Total is achieved by adding all of the subtotals in Column D.

To find the average level of participation, divide the Grand Total by the total number of activities, i.e. the total of Column D divided by the total of Column C is the average level of participation.

A leisure level scale is provided to gain information helpful in evaluating the participant's quality of leisure participation. Note that the more activities one has, the more potential for accuracy. The participant must list at least ten activities (positive and negative) to be sure the results are meaningful. Fewer than ten activities is indicative of either a problem with reporting or a problem with having too few leisure activities during a thirty day period.

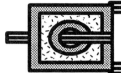 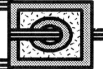

Step 3 Part B
Leisure Participation

Name _____   Date _____

A. Leisure Activities that I have participated in within the last 30 days	B. Leisure Level		C. Times I participated in the last 30 days		D. Activity Points
		X		=	
		X		=	
		X		=	
		X		=	
		X		=	
		X		=	
		X		=	
		X		=	
		X		=	
		X		=	
		X		=	
		X		=	
		X		=	
		X		=	
		X		=	
		X		=	
		X		=	
		X		=	
Totals for columns C and D					

Level of Participation: Total of Column D divided by Total of Column C _____

My thoughts about my level of participation ...

My feelings about how I spend my time are ...

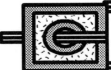

Step 3 Part B
Leisure Participation

A) List the leisure or recreation activities that you have participated in within the last 30 days, including positive and negative activities. List at least 10 activities.
B) Give each activity points from the Leisure Level Model.
C) Fill in how many times you have participated in each activity within the last 30 days.
D) Multiply column B times column C and put the answer in column D.
E) Count up the number of times you participated in activities in column C and put it at the bottom of column C.
F) Add or subtract in column D to get the total and put it at the bottom of column D.
G) Divide the total in column D by the total number of activities in column C to get your average level of participation shown in the chart below.

Leisure Participation Scale

Cathartic Level	Participation in at least one leisure activity with a great deal of emotional release. The event resulted in personal growth.
Level 4	Participation is creative, inventive, imaginative. Be cautious to not spend excessive time in your own world.
Level 2 to 4	Participation seems to be in balance and on a therapeutic level. Leisure pursuits are enjoyable, expressive, active and helpful in solving problems.
Level 1 to 2	Participation spectator. Be cautious that you don't let life pass you by. Also, negative/harmful activity participation can jeopardize the balance in your life.
Level 0	Participation co-dependent. You need to talk, trust, feel, think and live for yourself. Perhaps unhealthy, negative choices are highly influencing your behaviors.
Level -1 to -2	Participation harmful/hurting. These choices may seem fun and harmless but are often driven by anger or unmet needs. Leisure counseling and education can help you attain a higher leisure level or quality of life.
Lost Freedom	Counseling may be necessary to restoring you to a healthy, positive level of participation. Seek help, direction and support from a friend, family member, clergy or counselor. Freedom can be restored and it is worth the trouble.

Note: Quality of leisure is not just how many points you scored. Participation at a high level alone does not necessarily mean that you are enjoying yourself. Also you must not get discouraged with a low score. Since you control your own leisure choices, you can change toward healthy positive choices.

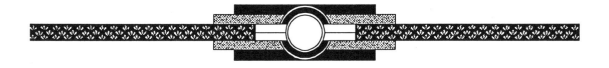

Part C: Leisure Attitude Awareness

Part C gives the participant the opportunity to explore his/her attitude of self and various aspects of leisure. If a participant is not aware of his/her thoughts, feelings and ideas (which , in turn, influence attitude), s/he will have difficulty improving the quality of his/her leisure. It is also valuable information for the staff in identifying the participant's outlook on his/her leisure lifestyle.

An attitude is a mental position, a state of mind, a perception. Many times attitude (slang) is thought to have a negative connotation, i.e., "you have an attitude" or "that attitude, is what's getting you in trouble." In this section attitude is used in the traditional sense. It may be positive, negative or neutral. Leisure participation is definitely affected by the participant's attitude and the participant's attitude toward life is definitely affected by the participant's leisure participation.

There are different theories regarding how people change their thoughts, feelings, beliefs, attitude, behavior; how they interact and which affects the other. Although the word attitude is not always mentioned, it is implied in the following. Rational-Emotive Therapy, based on the work of Albert Ellis, basically states that our feelings are caused more by our thoughts about events than by the events themselves. Our beliefs affect the way we feel about an event.

Dr. W. M. Glasser's Reality Therapy/Control Therapy Psychology defines behavior as what we do, what we think, most of what we feel and how our bodies behave. It proposes that the easiest of these to change is what we do and what we think. Change these and feelings and physiological responses will eventually change. Our attitudes are a sum of the internal pictures we have of how we see the outside world. To change our attitudes we need to change what we do or think. If that does not work, we need to modify the internal picture.

Charles Swindoll's popular view of attitude is

> The longer I live, the more I realize the impact of attitude on life. Attitude, to me, is more important than facts. It is more important than the pats, than education, than money, than circumstances, than failures, than successes, than what other people think or say or do. It is more important than appearance, giftedness or skill. It will make or break a company ... a church ... a home. The remarkable thing is we

have a choice every day regarding the attitude we will embrace for that day. We cannot change our past ... we cannot change the fact that people will act in a certain way. We cannot change the inevitable. The only thing we can do is play on the one string we have and that is our attitude ... I am convinced that life is 10% what happens to me and 90% how I react to it. And so it is with you ... we are in charge of our Attitudes.

Mihaly Csikszentmihaly[6] writes of happiness as not dependent on outside events, but how we interpret them:

What I "discovered" was that happiness is not something that happens. It is not the result of good fortune or random chance. It is not something that money can buy or power command. It does not depend on outside events, but rather, on how we interpret them. Happiness, in fact, is a condition that must be prepared for, cultivated and defended privately by each person. People who learn to control inner experience will be able to determine the quality of their lives, which is as close as any of us can come to being happy.

It is not the intention of this book to list all of the various theories of therapy, but to make you aware of the importance of attitude in leisure decision making. A goal in recreational therapy may be to help develop a positive healthy attitude through recreational therapy programming or Leisure Plan. A useful tool in assessing your participant's leisure attitude may be the (LAM) Leisure Attitude Measurement which reviews attitudes on the levels of 1) cognitive, 2) affective, 3) behavioral. Taken from the Idyll Arbor Leisure Battery.

The thirteen Leisure Awareness Stems[7] in the form on the next page, are related to the six functional domains of recreational therapy as shown in the chart below:

Recreational Therapy Domain	Question
leisure	4, 6, 11
physical	3, 8
cognitive	7, 13
daily living	10, 12
social	1, 2, 11
psychological	5, 9

Answers to the stems where the participant describes his/her thoughts, feelings and ideas, give insight into the participant's attitude toward life. This can be helpful in understanding your participant and giving direction to his/her leisure.

---

[6]Csikszentmihaly, M., 1990. **Flow: The Psychology of Optimal Experience**, p. 2. New York. Harper Perennial

[7]A "stem" is a sentence fragment that the participant finishes, for example, "When I have time alone, I feel ...".

Step 3 Part C
Leisure Attitude Awareness

Name _____   Date _____

Please complete each stem and write a brief explanation

1) Most important at a party or social engagement is ...

2) When I have time alone, I feel ...

3) When I think of physical activity and exercise, I ...

4) My free time at home is ...

5) I express myself best in recreation activities that I ...

6) I believe my leisure time would be more positive if ...

7) When I was younger, my attitude toward free time was ...

8) I like to keep in shape physically by ...

9) I believe what I do during my free time affects my self esteem because ...

10) When there is work needing to be done and I have free time, I think ...

11) My attitude toward my family doing leisure activities and spending time together is ...

12) I believe my accomplishments at work or school are enhanced by my leisure activities because ...

13) When I think of activities, where I have to use my brain I ...

My Thoughts —

My Feelings —

My Ideas —

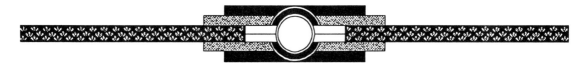

Part D: Days in My Life

Days In My Life is a quick and effective means for the participant to examine a typical 24 hour day. It includes both weekday and weekend categories as they may be very different. The therapist can look at the balance between work and leisure, identify amounts of sleep and rest, identify knowledge and understanding the participant has of how s/he spends his/her day and other pertinent information. Individual or group therapy can further reveal trouble areas such as when the participant is bored, lonely, getting high, having difficulty sleeping, etc. You can also identify high energy times, time available for healthy activities, time management ideas, etc.

Some participants have a problem with the idea of a "typical day" because they feel that all days are different. However in most cases the participant is able to identify patterns in his/her daily schedule that are typical of each day.

The following self awareness questions are helpful in exploring significant aspects of leisure and potential problems in how the participant spends his/her time.

MY THOUGHTS ABOUT:

1)   The amount of time I spend with my family ...
2)   The amount of sleep I get ...
3)   The amount of time I participate in healthy leisure activities ...
4)   The most positive thing I do with my time is ...
5)   I would like to change ...

Variations of this simple form can be made to gain other information and an understanding such as:

- The ideal or perfect day
- My day as a child (the child within)
- My day as an adult (for adolescents)
- A special day or event

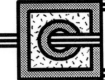 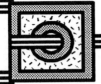

Step 3 Part D
Days In My Life

Name _____   Date _____

Fill in <u>specifically</u> how you spend your time in a typical 24 hour day.

Days In My Life	Weekday	Weekend
7:00 am	_____	_____
8:00 am	_____	_____
9:00 am	_____	_____
10:00 am	_____	_____
11:00 am	_____	_____
12:00 pm	_____	_____
1:00 pm	_____	_____
2:00 pm	_____	_____
3:00 pm	_____	_____
4:00 pm	_____	_____
5:00 pm	_____	_____
6:00 pm	_____	_____
7:00 pm	_____	_____
8:00 pm	_____	_____
9:00 pm	_____	_____
10:00 pm	_____	_____
11:00 pm	_____	_____
12:00 am	_____	_____
1:00 am	_____	_____
2:00 am	_____	_____
3:00 am	_____	_____
4:00 am	_____	_____
5:00 am	_____	_____
6:00 am	_____	_____

Step 3 Part D
Days In My Life

My thoughts about:

1) The amount of time I spend with my family ...

2) The amount of sleep I get ...

3) The amount of time I participate in healthy leisure activities ...

4) The most positive thing I do with my time is ...

5) I would like to change ...

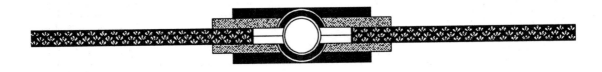

Part E: Leisure Resources

The leisure resources section consists of two parts: 1) a crossword puzzle with community and home resources and 2) a map and wide range list of community and surrounding area resources.

Many of our participants need to make changes in people, places and things to become healthy. In other words, if our participants continue to associate with the same people in the same situations, internal permanent change is nearly impossible. Knowledge of available resources is important for increasing the potential for lifestyle change. The crossword puzzle is an educational activity that includes various resources at home and within the community, along with your input into the resources available.

Community Resources

There are 11 community resource clues to solve in filling in the crossword puzzle. They are A through K and are generic resources found in most communities. The puzzle resources are down on the Leisure Resource Puzzle. The answers are as follows:
A) Chamber, B) ice skating, C) bowling, D) museum, E) zoo, F) golf, G) GED, H) walk,
I) concert, J) library, K) fitness.

Home Resources

Many people believe that in order to increase leisure participation they have to purchase a boat, a truck to pull it, a camper shell to sleep in. This of course is not true and this type of understanding of leisure deters the participant from participating in simple meaningful leisure activities. There are 11 home resource clues to solve in filling in the crossword puzzle. They are 1 through 11 and are resources that are pertinent to most home settings. The puzzle resources are across on the Leisure Resource Puzzle. The answers are as follows: 1) read, 2) garden, 3) hobby, 4) meditation, 5) cooking, 6) home, 7) pets, 8) games, 9) music, 10) social, 11) television.

Map and Community Resources

Following the Leisure Resource Puzzle is an excellent space to include a map of the participants community (telephone books usually work well), along with information about many various community resources. Include telephone numbers, addresses, bus routes and other helpful information. Most recreational therapy departments already have a community resources file available to the therapists. It is just a matter of putting it into a user friendly package for participant use. In smaller communities it may be helpful to put in other communities with different resources. Also helpful is a listing of **Emergency and Important Phone Numbers** including: your facility and similar facilities, 911 (or other) for emergency, AA, emergency room, department of social services, rape crisis center, support groups, etc.

Step 3 Part E
Crossword Puzzle

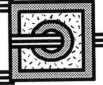

Community Resources — DOWN

A) This city resource has pamphlets and information of community events _____ of Commerce.

B) This activity requires a cold floor and funny shoes — 2 words.

C) This activity used to be called nine pins.

D) A place to go to learn of the past or the future and see important items, pictures and stories.

E) Here, I can study animals and observe them as they are in the wild.

F) This sport is getting more and more popular, probably due to the challenge, the beauty of the course and the walk that includes 18 holes.

G) If I did not get my high school diploma, I can attend classes and study to get these initials.

H) Depending upon the weather, I may go barefoot, need boots or wear comfortable shoes to participate in this aerobic activity. I could go with my neighbor or take my dog when I go for a _____.

I) I may see Aretha Franklin, Garth Brooks, Slayer, Pearl Jam or the local rap, rock or country group when I attend a music _____.

J) They have computers here and assistants to help me find information, where I can read and learn about just about anything.

K) Here, I can lift weights, go for a swim, join an aerobics class, play volleyball and shoot hoops. It is a _____ center.

Home Resources — ACROSS

1) I can easily keep up with current events on a daily basis or get lost in an adventure when I participate in this activity.

2) Indoors or outdoors I can watch my fruits flourish.

3) Model cars, sewing, woodwork, crafts, all make up having a _____.

4) It is best to be alone and in a quiet place for relaxation or _____.

5) Add a little bit of this and a little bit of that. I call this kitchen activity _____.

6) Many times this leisure time activity requires tools and elbow grease _____ maintenance.

7) These friends require much tender loving care and feeding.

8) Lets sit around the table or on the floor and play _____.

9) Sometimes this makes me relax and sometimes I dance, I may even sing.

10) Entertaining others or having your friends over to share a meal or fun is being _____.

11) Too much of this will steal away time from all of the other activities.

92

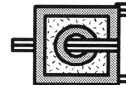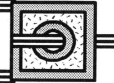

Step 3 Part E
Crossword Puzzle

Name _____   Date _____

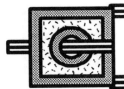
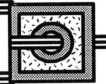

Step 3 Part E
Crossword Puzzle

Name _____   Date _____

^CB

³HOBBY

^AC
H
A   ^GG
B   E
⁴MEDITAT^BION
E   C
¹READ   ⁸GAMES

O
W
L
I
N
G

^DM   ^FG
U   O
⁷PETS   ¹⁰SOCIAL
K   F
²GARDEN

^HW   U
A   ⁹MUSIC   ^JL
L   N   I
^IC   T   B
⁵COOKING   R
O   A
N   ^KF   R
¹¹TELEVISION   Y
R   I
T   T
^EZ   N
⁶HOME S
O   S
S

94

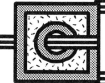

Step 3 Part E
Emergency Numbers

Service	Name of Agency	Phone Number
Emergency Services		**Dial 911**
Hospital		
Alcoholics Anonymous		
Mental Health Services		
Suicide Prevention		
Department of Social Services (day number)		
Department of Social Services (night number)		
Chemical Dependency Support Group		
Rape Crisis Center		
Frequently Called Numbers		

Step 3 Part E
Spectator & Entertainment

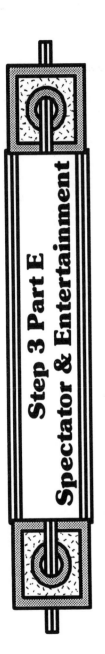

Activity	Facility	Address	Phone	Times	How to Get There	Other

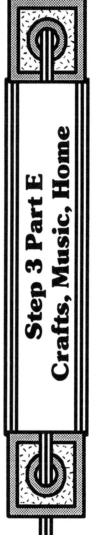

Step 3 Part E
Crafts, Music, Home

Activity	Facility	Address	Phone	Times	How to Get There	Other

97

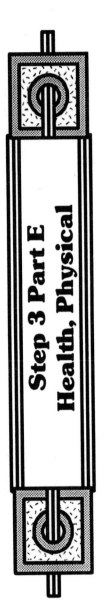

Step 3 Part E
Health, Physical

Activity	Facility	Address	Phone	Times	How to Get There	Other

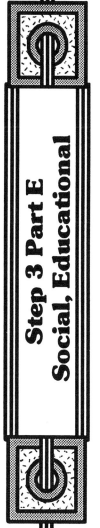

Step 3 Part E
Social, Educational

Activity	Facility	Address	Phone	Times	How to Get There	Other

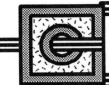 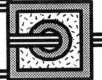

Step 3 Part E
Community Map

The therapist needs to place a map of the participant's local community on this page. It is recommended that the therapist also highlight, number or otherwise note the important leisure and health resource centers on the map for the participant. Use the bottom of this page to type in the names of the resource centers that are highlighted on the map.

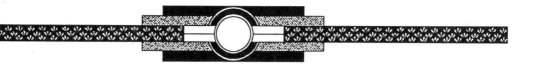

Part F: Things I Enjoy

This step is aimed at identifying pleasurable activities. The amount of pleasure the participant receives from leisure participation is affected by the status of the participant's mental health. The potential for pleasure decreases with decreased mental health. The opposite is also true. Increased pleasure in leisure participation will affect the participant's mental health in a positive direction. Note that pleasure in a healthy sense is defined as leisure activities on a healthy/positive level on the Leisure Level Model. This is not to be confused with pleasure seeking (which would actually be a lower level on the model).

Many participants that have been highly involved in drugs and alcohol or in exciting unhealthy leisure choices such as stealing or gang involvement may initially find simple leisure activities boring and not fun. It is important for the participant and the therapist to be aware of this for programming purposes and for the participant's leisure decision making. Adventure and high stimulus programming may be necessary to have a therapeutic impact for some participants. This should be followed by leisure counseling and education so that the participant will eventually be able to enjoy simple activities also. I often use an example of eating a hot pepper or spicy food which deadens the taste buds to milder food. Time away from the hot pepper will allow the taste buds to taste and enjoy the subtlety of milder food. In terms of leisure choices and enjoyment, time away from unhealthy negative choices will make way for enjoyment of positive healthy choices.

Some highly depressed participants are unable to receive enjoyment from pleasurable activities or have stopped participating in leisure activities due to their depression. An old recovery saying is "fake it till you make it". This is important as participants will often say "I don't feel like doing this activity" and most of the time really don't. It is important for them to understand that they may need to practice (many times) to relearn the process of enjoying leisure activity.

Things I enjoy, is broken down into four areas of leisure, i.e. A) spectator, entertainment, B) arts, crafts, music, drama, dance, home activities, C) exercise, games, sports, physical activities, health, D) education, cultural activities, collecting, volunteerism, social activities. These areas will be further addressed in Steps 7, 8, 9 and 10. Those steps are participatory, an extension to the educational aspects of these steps.

It is important for the participant to gain an understanding of what is enjoyable to him/her. Many of us do what we do without stopping to think whether we really enjoy it.

The categories of alone, family, friends will identify social aspects of each activity. The cost category will give monetary information, while the how often category will give information regarding the quantity of involvement for each activity. This information will be important in leisure counseling, making changes in lifestyle and in the participant's future leisure decision making.

If necessary, examples for each leisure area are given in Steps 7, 8, 9 and 10.

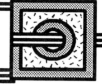

Step 3 Part F
Things I Enjoy

1)   Fill in 5 activities that you enjoy in each area.
2)   Place a check in the category to show who else participates in the activity with you.
3)   Fill in appropriate cost.
4)   Fill in how often you participate in the activity.

A)   Spectator, entertainment

activity	alone	family	friends	cost	how often
1.					
2.					
3.					
4.					
5.					

B)   Arts, crafts, music, drama, dance, home activities

activity	alone	family	friends	cost	how often
1.					
2.					
3.					
4.					
5.					

C)   Exercise, games, sports, physical activities, health

activity	alone	family	friends	cost	how often
1.					
2.					
3.					
4.					
5.					

D)   Educational, cultural, collecting, volunteerism, social activities

activity	alone	family	friends	cost	how often
1.					
2.					
3.					
4.					
5.					

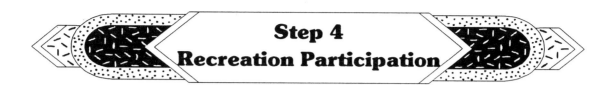

Step 4
Recreation Participation

Step 4 is the first of the participatory steps in the **Leisure Step Up** program. This step involves participation in four separate leisure activities, one in each of the four upper leisure levels. This step may take a week or more, depending upon the participant's leisure lifestyle. The participant should not put activities down that have previously been done but activities that the participant does after completing Step 3. The date, time and length are significant in helping the participant identify leisure planning in Step 6.

The participant then writes a brief paragraph about each activity. It may be important to point out the significance of the activities that the participant chooses to participate in, i.e. are the choices different than the choices prior to beginning the **Leisure Step Up Workbook**? Note that this step allows for no participation in unhealthy/negative choices.

105

Step 4
Recreation Participation

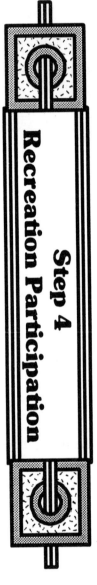

This step is participatory as opposed to educational. You actively do something. Participate in at least one leisure activity in each of the four leisure levels (1, 2, 3, 4). There is NO participation in the unhealthy, negative levels. To be sure that you understand the meaning of the four positive levels, review the chart of the levels shown in Step 3.

For each activity, write the type of activity, the date and time you did the activity and the amount of time you participated.

Level	Activity	Date	Time	Length	Description of what you did and what you felt
4					
3					
2					
1					

106

Step 5
Leisure of the Past

In psychotherapy, dealing with past issues and resolution (letting go) of those past issues is an essential step toward a new healthy life. How issues are resolved depends on the issues and the individual. For example, dealing with past issues for a psychotic individual would need to be handled with extensive sensitivity and communication coordinated with the treatment team. Dealing with a teenager who is defiant may need to be from a confrontive positive position. In any case, problems with leisure choices coincide with other problem areas in the participant's life.

Many individuals started drug or alcohol use about the same time their parents divorced or when they suffered another loss. Many participants stopped healthy leisure participation because they were under severe stress. The participant needs to learn that especially at problematic times in his/her life, participating in healthy, positive leisure can be a significant factor in getting through the problem period.

Leisure of the past identifies both unhealthy and healthy participation of the near and distant past. Most participants have little trouble finding significant periods in their lives when they made unhealthy and healthy choices. The emotions connected with these times may be intense enough to require individual or group therapy before the experiences can be written down as part of this step. Even if therapy is not required before this exercise, the participant is still asked to share this step with a counselor or in a group therapy session after it is completed.

This exercise helps the participant identify a time frame for past leisure choices, other aspects of life within that time frame and social aspects regarding the specific leisure choices listed. The Stem ("My feelings about my past leisure participants are ...") allows the participant to write down feelings regarding his/her past. This may give direction for the therapist/counselor in helping the participant deal with and express his/her feelings.

The question ("Would I be better off if I changed my lifestyle?") looks at the commitment of the participant regarding past leisure choice prior to Step 6, Leisure of the Future.

The question ("Does anything now prevent me from healthy positive participation?") addresses barriers which the participant will need to overcome to reach a higher functioning leisure level.

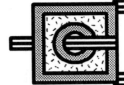 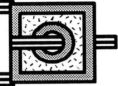

Step 5
Leisure of the Past

Name _____   Date _____

List significant or important leisure activities that you have participated in the past. Put Unhealthy Negative Choices, including Levels Lost Freedom, -1 and -2 on the second page and Healthy Positive Choices including Levels 1, 2, 3, 4 and Cathartic Level on the third page. Answer these questions for each activity:

- What leisure level was I participating on?
- When did I start and stop these activities?
- What was going on in my life at the time?
- Who got me into or out of these activities?

Also answer the questions on the fourth page.
When you are finished, share Step 5 with a counselor or in a group therapy session.

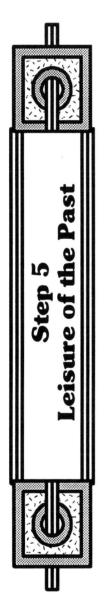

Step 5
Leisure of the Past

Unhealthy Choices

Activity Choice	Level	Start	Stop	What was going on?	Who got me involved?

109

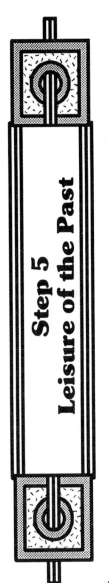

Step 5
Leisure of the Past

Healthy Choices

Activity Choice	Level	Start	Stop	What was going on?	Who got me involved?

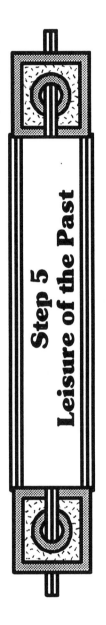

Step 5
Leisure of the Past

My feelings about my past leisure participation are ...

Would I be better off if I changed my lifestyle? Why?

Does anything now prevent me from healthy positive participation?

111

Step 6
Leisure of the Future

Spontaneity in leisure is great and is essential in a holistic approach to leisure participation. However, total reliance upon spontaneity will generally result in lack of structure in the participant's leisure lifestyle and may lead to unhealthy negative leisure participation.

It is essential to plan ahead. This does not mean we don't live in the present; it simply means that we need to plan, so that we can enjoy living that one day at a time. In looking at the leisure planning process, we actually begin enjoying the leisure activity during the planning stage. So the therapy begins during the planning stage and continues through the reminiscing aspects of the activity.

Many of our participants run away from feelings and problems through substance abuse, physical problems, rage, inappropriate leisure choices, actually running away, etc. Many healthy people also run away from feelings and problems by appropriate leisure choices such as a weekend break, (mini) vacation or extended lunch. Vacations, movies, exercise, crafts, sports, etc. are at times an escape from daily stress and other problems.

One major difference between the two methods of escaping is that negative leisure activities create new problems without resolving the old ones while healthy escape allows the participant to face the problem rejuvenated, energetic and, perhaps, with a clearer understanding. Leisure is positive when it helps solve problems and negative when it makes them worse.

Step 6, Leisure of the Future, helps the participant plan future leisure activities which will create positive changes in his/her life. It includes:

1) listing the activity
2) estimating the cost
3) choosing a specific date and time
4) choosing who to go with
5) special needs or training
6) benefits of participation
7) barriers and adaptations

It is not necessary that the participant follow through with this exact plan, but the planning will serve as a guide for future planning and enhance the participant's ability to replan an activity if problems come up.

When the participant finishes the plan, you should help him/her go over it and note changes that need to be made.

Name _____   Date _____

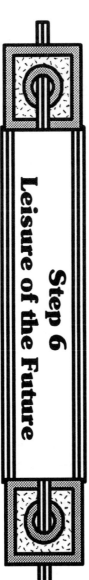

Step 6
Leisure of the Future

List five Leisure Interests with a specific plan for each. When you are finished, go over these plans with your counselor and note any changes that need to be made.

Activity	Time	Cost	With Whom?	Training	Benefits	Barriers

Is there anything that might prevent these activities from taking place?

Step 7
Community Participation

Step 7 begins active participation. The participant now puts knowledge and skills to the test by deciding how to spend his/her leisure time. This phase is important as it validates that the participant can do what s/he says s/he wants to do. The participant selects an activity to attend as a spectator.

Many of us have little difficulty associated with leisure participation within the community. Some participants however, become stressed, anxious or even have an extreme fear of community leisure participation. Being out of his/her home, being around others in crowds, having little knowledge of the community, lacking self trust or trust of others, may cause problems with this step. It is important for the participant to deal with stress, anxiety and fears before and after the activity to overcome barriers. This will allow freedom for future independent choices and functioning.

Mild to moderately depressed participants have a tendency to be isolated, withdrawn, lacking in motivation, energy, pleasures, interest and other various symptoms affecting participation in this step. Community leisure participation can act as a catalyst in helping the participant in psychotherapy and in other interventions by affecting these symptoms in a positive manner.

In this step the participant writes about the community experience, shares it with a counselor or in a group therapy, then writes his/her thoughts and feelings about the activity.

The participant may refer to Step 3, Part F for interest areas in spectator/entertainment activities. See the list below for examples.

Community Spectator, Entertainment

WATCHING:	ATTENDING:
Football	Fairs
Baseball	Car shows
Basketball	Art shows
Ballet	Carnivals
Plays	Museums
Musicians	Lectures
Comedians	Movies
Singers	Concerts

115

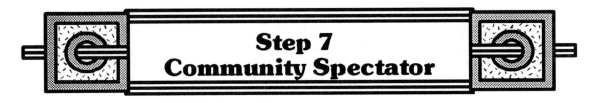

Step 7
Community Spectator

Name _____ Date _____

Participate as a spectator within the community. Write about the experience, share it with a counselor or in group therapy.

What was the activity?

My **thoughts** about the activity ...

My **feelings** about the activity ...

Will I do it again? Why?

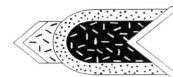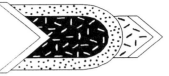

Step 8
Expressive Leisure
Participation

Step 8 includes activities in the areas of arts, crafts, music, drama, dance and home. These areas are generally thought of as highly expressive. Self expression is extremely important when the participant has difficulty verbalizing or has deep seated problems or secrets. Self expression is also important in dealing with stress, self awareness, anger and other significant aspects of mental health. This step allows the participant to enhance self esteem by seeing accomplishment in these areas.

Participation in arts, crafts, music, drama, dance and home activities are a part of all cultures and are as old as time itself. There is always something around the home to tinker with and fix. "The list", as we sometimes call it, can be a rewarding experience. From doodling to mechanical drawing, art is a means of controlling and putting things into perspective or showing them as we want them to be. Craft work involves a tactile experience putting creativity and skill together. Music has the power to energize or relax. It is a means of communication of who and what we are whether we create or just listen. Drama offers a means of vicariously living an aspect of our life, saying what we wish we could say, being who we wish we could be and then coming back to reality with a new life experience. Dance is a socially acceptable means of physical and emotional expression.

Two activity sheets are included in Step 8. The participant is to participate in two separate activities in different expressive areas. This allows the participant to experience various aspects of self expression, accomplishment and other benefits. The participant then writes about the experiences, thoughts, feelings and answers if they will participate in them again. It is important to share this step to problem solve and share the positive aspects of the activities.

The participant may refer to Step 3, Part F for his/her interests in these areas. See the following page for examples.

117

Expressive Leisure Activities

Arts	Crafts	Music	Drama	Dance	Home
drawing	leather	listening	movies	social dance	car repair
painting	pottery	instrument	plays	square dance	indoor plants
sketching	ceramics	singing	stories	rap dance	gardening
clay	sewing	reading music	skits	modern dance	baking
sculpting	knitting	writing music	puppets	dance aerobics	cooking
photography	wood work				pets
printing	models				picnics
					barbecue
					decorating
					furniture repair
					carpentry
					shopping

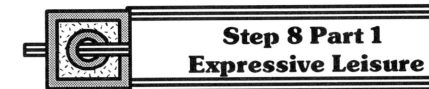 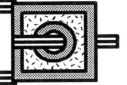

Step 8 Part 1
Expressive Leisure

Name _____ Date _____

Participate in an expressive leisure activity in the areas of arts, crafts, music, drama, dance and home activities. Activity 1 and Activity 2 should be in different areas. Write about the experience. Share it with a counselor or in group therapy.

What was the activity?

My **thoughts** about the activity ...

My **feelings** about the activity ...

Will I do it again? Why?

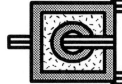

Step 8 Part 2
Expressive Leisure

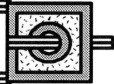

Name _____ Date _____

Participate in an expressive leisure activity in the areas of arts, crafts, music, drama, dance and home activities. Activity 1 and Activity 2 should be in different areas. Write about the experience. Share it with a counselor or in group therapy.

What was the activity?

My **thoughts** about the activity ...

My **feelings** about the activity ...

Will I do it again? Why?

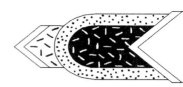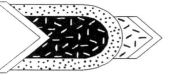

Step 9
Physical Leisure
Participation

Step 9 includes activities in the areas of exercise, games, sports, physical activity and health. Most therapists acknowledge that participation of a physical action is extremely therapeutic and beneficial. A social worker once told a group of hospital administrators, physicians and nurses that if 90% of the clients that he sees were involved in a structured exercise routine, they would not need his services. I believe that may be an exaggeration, but he believed it. I cannot over emphasize the importance of appropriate physical activity and exercise in becoming healthy. I find it necessary to give this area some attention since it is a necessary aspect of recreational therapy treatment and many mental health therapists look at physical activity and exercise as recreational therapy's only mode of treatment (far from the truth).

Therapeutic exercise is a term used for structured, goal oriented and prescribed activity or exercise of a physical nature which brings about a desired change in health. All activity and recreational therapy service programs should encompass some form of therapeutic exercise program. Some basic mental health benefits of therapeutic exercise include:

- Upright, open posture in stretching (opposite that of a closed, depressed posture)
- Stress reduction through deep breathing, tightening, relaxing and warming of muscles
- Empowerment of the participant to make healthy changes by his/her own participation
- Decreased symptoms of eating disorders by education and appropriate exercise patterns
- Decreased insomnia and poor sleep
- Increased motivation and energy
- Outlet for tension, aggression, anger and rage
- Decreased anxiety and fears
- Increased concentration, focus and alertness
- Decreased depression by increasing catecholamines (neurochemicals) in the brain
- Elevated mood by secreting endorphins into the blood system
- Decreased craving and less chance of relapse into drug and alcohol abuse
- Concrete goals and boundaries (without the possibility of manipulation) for the oppositional defiant/sociopath
- Increased positive social networking and a healthy place to attend (health club, youth club, sport, etc.)
- Understanding of failure and success in competition and play
- Understanding of fairness, cooperation and sportsmanship in team play
- Alternative positive leisure coping mechanisms
- Personal internal emotional strength and stamina as a metaphor to development of physical strength and stamina
- Enhancement of psychopharmacological therapy by enhancing the natural physiological response

- Positive attitude and outlook by the enhancement of the participant's general health
- Decreased anhedonia (inability to experience pleasure)
- Positive diversion from overwhelming problems
- Leader, follower and assertiveness skills in team play

Care and caution need to be used when involving participants in a therapeutic exercise program. Many participants have been inactive for years and need a slow introduction into therapeutic exercise. Work closely with the physician and treatment team to gain perspective into each participant's limitations and abilities. A fitness evaluation to determine body fat, cardiovascular efficiency, strength, endurance and flexibility may also be helpful. Proper leisure counseling will enhance the potential for post discharge participation. The following step analysis may be helpful in the development of an active leisure lifestyle.

Step analysis of beginning an exercise routine

Step	Cause
1. Lack of desire	due to lack of experience, fear, denial of need, etc.
2. Need arises to improve health	high cholesterol, feeling depressed, high blood pressure
3. Initial interest and motivation	due to health, weight, confrontation, peer pressure, etc.
4. Person researches	learns of exercise resources, gains self awareness and insight
5. Motivation born	person looks at various means of exercise and person participates
6. Various excuses	feeling sore in muscles, it didn't make a difference, I'm too old, fat, clumsy, etc. Continues or returns to step 1.
7. Person inspired	having a greater insight of self and exercise resources
8. Person participates	increasing in regularity. Continues or has sophisticated excuses and returns to step 1.
9. If continued regularly	person begins to experience benefits, increased energy, increased sleep, decreased depression, increased physical health, decreased fat, increased self-esteem, increased clear thinking, etc. Continued need for motivation, perhaps from an outside source. Participation somewhat difficult to initiate
10. Regular participation	truly enjoys exercise and activity, needs no motivation outside of activity, receives full benefits, complete lifestyle change

In Step 9, the participant is to participate in two activities in different leisure areas of exercise, games, sports, physical activity or health. They then write about the experience and share with a counselor or in group therapy. They should include thoughts and feelings and discuss future participation in this activity.

Two sheets are included, one for each separate leisure area. The participant may review his/her interests in Step 9 areas by referring back to Step 3, Part F. See the chart below for examples.

Physical Leisure Activities

Exercise	Games	Sports	Physical Activities	Health
weight training	horse shoes	bowling	horse riding	AA
jogging, running	miniature golf	softball	hunting	Alanon
relaxation therapy	Frisbee golf	golf	fishing	_____ teams
swimming	ping pong	skiing	bicycle riding	weight watcher
aerobics	tag	football	camping	
floor exercise	catch	baseball	hiking	
water aerobics		tennis	self defense	
stretching		volleyball	mountaineering	
step aerobics		basketball	ice skating	
walking			roller skating, roller blading	
			bird watching	

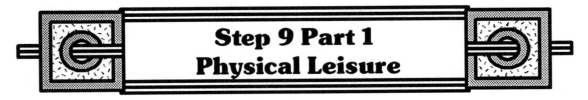

Step 9 Part 1
Physical Leisure

Name _____   Date _____

Participate in a physical leisure activity in the areas of exercise, games, sports, health or physical activities. Activity 1 and Activity 2 should be in different areas. Write about the experience. Share it with a counselor or in group therapy.

What was the activity?

My **thoughts** about the activity ...

My **feelings** about the activity ...

Will I do it again? Why?

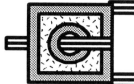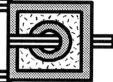

Step 9 Part 2
Physical Leisure

Name _____ Date _____

Participate in a physical leisure activity in the areas of exercise, games, sports, health or physical activities. Activity 1 and Activity 2 should be in different areas. Write about the experience. Share it with a counselor or in group therapy.

What was the activity?

My **thoughts** about the activity ...

My **feelings** about the activity ...

Will I do it again? Why?

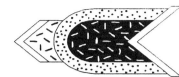 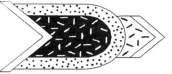

Step 10
Cultural Leisure
Participation

Step 10 include activities in the areas of education, culture, volunteerism, socializing and collecting. These activities all serve the purpose of bringing the participant out of him/herself and into contact with others.

Social activity offers essential opportunities to create and build relationships with others. Often the participant needs to avoid people, places and things that created problems in the past. Relating well with family and friends to build a support system for healthy choices is extremely important aspect of becoming and staying healthy. Step 10 includes leisure participation of a social nature. As a therapist, it is important to evaluate the participant's choices of leisure, making sure social aspects are in place. I have heard the following sad words from too many participants, "I have no friends." Friends who can support the participant in making healthy choices are important.

Have you ever stopped to think where our world would be without volunteers? Giving of our time is giving of our most valuable resource. There are however intrinsic rewards from volunteerism and service to others that place volunteer work on a high leisure level. Some of our participants no longer fit into the occupational model but still need to be productive members of society. Volunteerism is a unique way to feel wanted, accepted and to make a contribution that counts. Co-dependency issues may need to be dealt with regarding doing for others.

It is amazing what some people collect. Then again, what is important to one is not necessarily important to another. Collecting things is a popular way to spend leisure time, i.e. trading baseball and other cards, Elvis stamps, ball caps, CDs and coins.

It is difficult to say when an activity is educational since most activities have an educational component. Educational for the purpose of this step refer to those activities with the main focus on learning. There are many appropriate self help books, activities and video tapes available for the participant to explore personal growth.

Cultural activities seem to help us find the roots of being human. They connect individuals together with groups and teach us about the vastness of life. Cultural activities give us tradition, educating us about our importance.

In Step 10, the participant is involved in two activities in different areas of education, cultural, volunteerism, socializing or collecting. S/he writes about the experience and shares with a counselor or in group therapy, including thoughts, feelings and if they plan on participating in this activity again. The participant many refer to Step 3, Part F to review his/her interests in the above areas. See the following page for examples.

Cultural Leisure Activities

Educational	Cultural	Collecting	Volunteering	Social
reading	traveling	coins	nursing homes	church work
writing	church	cups	YMCA/YWCA	clubs
self help	choir	hats	hospitals	visiting
poetry	concerts	CDs	service groups	dating
	museums	tapes	youth groups	family leisure
	vacations	stamps	youth leagues	table games
	ethnic groups	cards	animal shelters	chess
		art	political campaigns	checkers
		antiques	environmental groups	card games
		rocks		pool

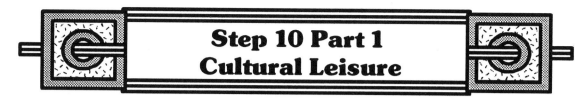

Name _____   Date _____

Participate in a cultural leisure activity in the areas of education, culture, collecting, volunteering or socializing. Activity 1 and Activity 2 should be in different areas. Write about the experience. Share it with a counselor or in group therapy.

What was the activity?

My **thoughts** about the activity ...

My **feelings** about the activity ...

Will I do it again? Why?

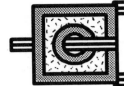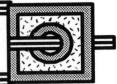

Step 10 Part 2
Cultural Leisure

Name _____ Date _____

Participate in a cultural leisure activity in the areas of education, culture, collecting, volunteering or socializing. Activity 1 and Activity 2 should be in different areas. Write about the experience. Share it with a counselor or in group therapy.

What was the activity?

My **thoughts** about the activity ...

My **feelings** about the activity ...

Will I do it again? Why?

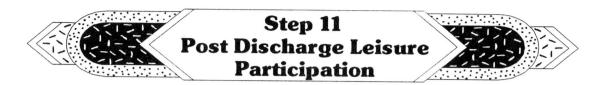

Step 11
Post Discharge Leisure Participation

Step 11 is the final step of the **Leisure Step Up Workbook**. It begins with Part A, a congratulations. Completing this workbook is quite an accomplishment and deserves a proper reward.

The participant is now ready to choose his/her own time, place and activity. With total freedom comes total benefit or consequence, whichever the choice may be. The participant is encouraged to share his/her leisure experiences with family, friends and others within his/her community.

Step 11, Part B, is an exercise similar to Step 3, Part B. The participant fills out the assignment to re-evaluate his/her leisure participation level. This time, the participant fills out the assignment on a daily basis for the next 30 days. At the end of 30 days, s/he calculates his/her level of participation and compares participation levels of Step 3 and Step 11.

If the participant is discharged prior to completion of the book, s/he may take the remaining steps and complete them on his/her own. If the participant remains within the facility after finishing the leisure workbook, s/he may participate in unit programming and in the recreation participation phase of the workbook.

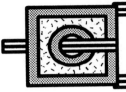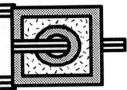

Step 11: Post Discharge Leisure Participation

Name _____   Date _____

Congratulations!!!

You are free and ready to participate in recreation activities of your own choice, time and place!!

I choose to ...

Write about your experiences and share it with family, friends and others!

Step 11: Post Discharge Leisure Participation Level

Name _____   Date _____

A. Leisure Activities that I have participated in within the last 30 days	B. Leisure Level		C. Times I participated in the last 30 days		D. Activity Points
		X		=	
		X		=	
		X		=	
		X		=	
		X		=	
		X		=	
		X		=	
		X		=	
		X		=	
		X		=	
		X		=	
		X		=	
		X		=	
		X		=	
		X		=	
		X		=	
		X		=	
		X		=	
Totals for columns C and D					

Level of Participation: Total of Column D / Total of Column C _____

Circle the best answer concerning the use of your leisure time
1. It is excellent and needs no changing.
2. I enjoy my leisure time but it needs minor changes.
3. I am aware of the changes I need to make and feel confident I will make them.
4. I will need some assistance with my leisure participation.
5. I need to review steps of the **Leisure Step Up Workbook** beginning with Step ___.

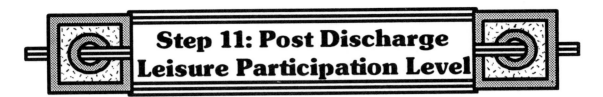

Step 11: Post Discharge Leisure Participation Level

A) Start today and keep track (on a daily basis) of all leisure activities that you participate in for the next 30 days.
B) Give each activity points from the Leisure Level Model.
C) Fill in how many times you participate in each activity.
D) Multiply column B times column C and put the answer in column D.
E) Count up the number of times you participated in activities in column C and put it at the bottom of column C.
F) Add or subtract in column D to get the total and put it at the bottom of column D.
G) Divide the total in column D by the total number of activities in column C to get your average level of participation shown in the chart below.

Leisure Participation Scale

Cathartic Level	Participation in at least one leisure activity with a great deal of emotional release. The event resulted in personal growth.
Level 4	Participation is creative, inventive, imaginative. Be cautious to not spend excessive time in your own world.
Level 2 to 4	Participation seems to be in balance and on a therapeutic level. Leisure pursuits are enjoyable, expressive, active and helpful in solving problems.
Level 1 to 2	Participation spectator. Be cautious that you don't let life pass you by. Also, negative/harmful activity participation can jeopardize the balance in your life.
Level 0	Participation co-dependent. You need to talk, trust, feel, think and live for yourself. Perhaps unhealthy, negative choices are highly influencing your behaviors.
Level -1 to -2	Participation harmful/hurting. These choices may seem fun and harmless but are often driven by anger or unmet needs. Leisure counseling and education can help you attain a higher leisure level or quality of life.
LOST FREEDOM	Counseling may be necessary to restoring you to a healthy, positive level of participation. Seek help, direction and support from a friend, family member, clergy or counselor. Freedom can be restored and it is worth the trouble.

Note: Quality of leisure is not just how many points you scored. Participation at a high level alone does not necessarily mean that you are enjoying yourself. Also you must not get discouraged with a low score. Since you control your own leisure choices, you can change toward healthy positive choices.